MERCURY, MISERY, AND ME

The Shocking Discovery That Cured My Chronic Fatigue Syndrome

Donna Haggerty

ISBN 978-1-63885-955-0 (Paperback)
ISBN 978-1-63885-956-7 (Digital)

Copyright © 2022 Donna Haggerty
All rights reserved
First Edition

This book should not be regarded as a guide to self-diagnosis, self-treatment, or a proven cure. The cooperation of a healthcare professional is essential to the principles and techniques discussed in this book.

All rights reserved. No part of this publication may be reproduced, distributed, or transmitted in any form or by any means, including photocopying, recording, or other electronic or mechanical methods without the prior written permission of the publisher. For permission requests, solicit the publisher via the address below.

Covenant Books
11661 Hwy 707
Murrells Inlet, SC 29576
www.covenantbooks.com

I have dedicated this book to give hope, especially for those who have suffered for years just like I did. I found the answers to heal myself from what I was being forced to believe was incurable. I want to share my discovery and the newfound awareness that restored me to good health once again.

1. Do you feel like you have been short-changed by the medical field?
2. Do you feel hopeless from being told by the medical profession that there is no cure for chronic fatigue syndrome?
3. Have you tried every treatment and drug possible to heal yourself, thinking that this one was the answer, only to be let down once again?

I wrote this book to provide hope to millions of people, like myself, who have been told by the professional field that there is no cure for autoimmune diseases.

I feared my destiny until I learned that I had
the power to change my health and life.

—Unknown

CONTENTS

I wanted you to see what real courage is, instead of getting
the idea that courage is a man with a gun in his hand. It's
when you know you're licked before you begin but you
begin anyway and you see it through no matter what.

—Harper Lee, *To Kill a Mockingbird,* 1960

If we do not change our direction, we are
likely to end up where we are headed.

—Ancient Chinese proverb

ACKNOWLEDGMENTS

I want to thank Dr. Hal Huggins who was the first toxicity of amalgams, better known as silver fillings, consequently showing so much concern for humanity.

I find Dr. Huggins to be a brave and loving individual, so willing to risk criticism and the potential loss of his license in order to protect the welfare of his patients and safeguard public health.

If it wasn't for Dr. Huggins writing of the most shocking, awakening, and scientific evidence about silver fillings in his book *It's All in Your Head*, I wouldn't be alive today. Thank you, Dr. Huggins. My love goes out to you for saving my life. I hope to have the opportunity and honor to meet you someday!

Dr. Huggins has been practicing dentistry for over thirty years using a multidisciplinary approach to treat the toxicity found in dental patients. He now travels around the world helping to develop centers that offer cures using his nontoxic approach. Dr. Huggins has several books and videos that can be purchased on the internet at www.hugnet.com.

I would like to thank Dr. Richard Saitta for being so positive and giving me so much hope. He kept me alive while I was searching for the answers to the enigma that was poisoning my body and causing the debilitating illness of chronic fatigue syndrome. He is such a very loving, dedicated, and open-minded medical doctor.

Dr. Saitta is a role model for other doctors. By promoting greater self-alliance and self-awareness, he uses his most valuable and personal resources to protect the health of our society.

Dr. Saitta was born in Italy and grew up in France. Besides being a medical doctor, he expanded his medical knowledge by studying and learning about herbal medicine and acupuncture in China. He offers hair mineral analysis testing to detect heavy metals in the body and chelation therapy for their detoxification. Dr. Saitta practices in Marco Island, Florida, and Naples, Florida.

I also want to recognize my dear and beautiful children—Tara, Shanna, and Sean—for their love, support, and all of the special things they did to encourage me to fight for my health and make me feel so special. To my daughter Shanna, thank you for never leaving my side and keeping such a positive attitude while encouraging me to fight for my life every day. My three children have and always will be the light of my life.

THERE IS THE RISK YOU CANNOT AFFORD TO TAKE AND THERE IS THE RISK YOU CANNOT AFFORD NOT TO TAKE.

—Peter Drucker

INTRODUCTION

I am not a medical doctor, dentist, or scientist. I am a human being who suffered for fourteen years, bedridden with chronic fatigue syndrome.

Traveling from state to state, I visited every medical doctor, holistic practitioner, and treatment center that I thought might cure me and restore my health.

I am very pleased and excited to share the discovery and my newfound awareness. The metals that most of us are exposed to every day had a poisoning effect on me. They caused what seemed like a lifetime of anguish, sorrow, and despair while forcing me to live with a chronic and devastating illness.

I am sure that you, as I, had no idea that the metals placed inside your mouth by your trusted dentist could ruin your health and destroy your well-being.

After reading my book, you will be aware of my discovery that will enable you to lay the stepping-stones on your path to wellness.

In Chapter 42, I've listed the steps that brought me to wellness. You may choose to follow them as you please. Our health depends on us, and only we can make the choice to change, as needed, to recover from chronic fatigue syndrome.

GOD, GRANT ME THE SERENITY TO ACCEPT THE THINGS I
CANNOT CHANGE, THE COURAGE TO CHANGE THE THINGS
I CAN, AND THE WISDOM TO KNOW THE DIFFERENCE.
—The Serenity Prayer

REAL KNOWLEDGE IS TO KNOW THE EXTENT OF ONE'S IGNORANCE.
—Confucius

1

Chronic Fatigue Syndrome

I don't know what you have read or been told by the medical field about chronic fatigue syndrome, if anything. However, I am so delighted to share what I learned about this devasting and overwhelming illness. Probably the most frightful and devastating episode in my life was being told by the medical profession that there isn't a cure and that they have not discovered any drugs to eliminate the symptoms.

I was told that chronic fatigue syndrome is similar to mononucleosis, having no known cause. Common symptoms are long-term and low-grade fever, headache, recurring sore throat, upper respiratory infection, fatigue, lymph node swelling, intestinal problems, muscle-and-joint pain, irritability, mood swings, anxiety, depression, temporary memory loss, and sleep disturbances. I don't know what symptoms you are experiencing, but I was unfortunate enough to have suffered with every one and more.

There is hope! I do not have chronic fatigue syndrome today! All the upsetting and stressful symptoms that destroyed most of my life have become only a memory.

CHRONIC

1. Lasting a long time or recurring.
2. Having an ailment. *(Webster's Dictionary)*

FATIGUE

The decreased capacity or complete inability of an organism, an organ, or a part to function normally; because of excessive stimulation or prolonged exertion. *(American Heritage Dictionary)*

SYNDROME

1. A group of symptoms that collectively indicate or characterize a disease, psychological disorder, or other abnormal condition.
2. A complex of symptoms indicating the existence of an undesirable condition or quality.
3. A distinctive or characteristic pattern of behavior. *(American Heritage Dictionary)*

The symptoms that disappeared after the removal of metals in my mouth were as follows:

1. Chronic fatigue
2. Stomach feeling raw
3. Unexplained intestinal pain
4. Constant pain in legs
5. Severe anemia
6. Excessive itching of skin
7. Unexplained ulcers
8. Constant metallic taste in mouth

9. Severe bleeding of gums
10. Swollen liver
11. Severe depression
12. Suicidal thoughts
13. Confusion
14. Tremors of the body
15. Frequent diarrhea
16. Severe phobias
17. Severe weakness
18. Lungs felt as if they were bleeding
19. Brain felt as if it was bleeding
20. Totally bedridden
21. Frequent headaches
22. Neck pain
23. Swollen lymph nodes
24. Flu-like symptoms
25. Constant joint pain
26. Irritability
27. Bloated feeling throughout my body
28. Constant upper respiratory infections
29. Severe dehydration
30. Blurred vision and dry eyes

2

My Dentist Poisoned Me

It can't be called malpractice. The American Dental Association, our noble and trusted medical society, founded by dentists close to one hundred fifty years ago, states that it is impossible for silver fillings or any other metals to have any side effects on a human being. In my case, they couldn't be more wrong. If the ADA had only started to protect us and reveal the truth, there would probably be more lawsuits than the entire criminal justice system or even the universe could handle. Most importantly, many diseases, I'm sure, would be eliminated.

I hope that the American Dental Association fully understands that fourteen years of my life were taken away from me, replaced by severe mental anguish, physical suffering, and almost the loss of my life.

During this time, my three children suffered with mental anguish and were emotionally drained as this happened during a very critical stage of their lives. It had been virtually impossible to obtain health insurance from any company due to my extensive medical record. I lost thousands upon thousands of dollars, including my home and automobile. Finally, after fourteen years of desolation, I discovered what was killing me and causing chronic fatigue syndrome. I lost everything except for my life, which I managed to save.

My perception of doctors, dentists, and the medical field has changed. Although these professionals appear to be godlike, they are just mortals like you and me. Yes, they have gone through many more years of education than most and were compelled to labor under the guidance of those more knowledgeable, as interns, before justifiably deserving to be treated as idols, earning more money. However, the facts remain clear: They are not perfect.

3

Wake Up, America!

We the people need to speak out! This is the only way that our government will listen! I am sure that millions of people are being poisoned every day, year after year.

Yes, my dear dentist is the last person I would have accused of making me deathly ill.

Unknown to me, I was continuously and slowly consuming one of the most poisonous substances known to man. My body was accumulating a material that we are warned not to touch. Who would ever think it could be possible to have poisonous toxic materials in your teeth?

MERCURY

1. A heavy silver white HIGHLY TOXIC metallic element.
2. The only one that is liquid at room temperature. *(Webster's Dictionary)*

4

Shocking Poison!

After fourteen years of suffering, I was finally introduced to compu-tron testing and two books titled *It's All in Your Head* and *The Cure for All Diseases*. I now learned that the metals in my mouth were poisoning me every hour of the day and causing my serious health problems. These two books were extremely convincing, and I highly recommend reading them.

My precious silver fillings were not all silver, possibly 50 percent or more were mercury. My crowns weren't 100 percent porcelain either. Only the outside was porcelain; the inside of the crowns was gray in color, being another form of metal, nickel, and aluminum.

At one time, I had the impression that my crowns were 100 percent porcelain due to the heavy price tag. I was never informed differently. Why didn't the dentist tell me that the inside of the crowns were made up of different materials and that my fillings contained mercury, a poison? The FDA requires manufacturers to inform the public of the ingredients found in food, alcohol, drugs, and of the cancer-causing ingredients found in tobacco. Why shouldn't dentists be mandated by law to report the materials they are permanently placing in our mouths as well? If food, plants, animals, and other inert substances like dust or molds can be life-threatening to some sensitive and allergic people, why don't dentists realize that metals can be just as serious?

Sorry, Mr. Dentist, but I don't think that I would have been very pleased if you had informed me that you were placing aluminum and nickel in my mouth. Of course, if I was informed that mercury was used in my silver fillings, I would have told you that you were crazy and would have never let you place a known poisonous metal in my mouth. Unfortunately, I was never informed or given the option of using any other type of filling, such as composite (white) fillings. You just went ahead and used the amalgam (silver) fillings.

Why wasn't I given a choice? Do most people who are given a choice between the white (composite) or gray (silver) fillings think that the only significant reason for this option is for personal appearance or financial savings? Do you think that people would be able to make a wiser selection if they were given the choice of poisonous or nonpoisonous fillings?

In medicine, if a drug has one chance in a thousand of causing an adverse reaction, the patient is informed. I have learned that a dentist may place any number of substances listed as toxic by the Environmental Protection Agency (EPA) in their patients' mouths without giving the slightest hint of the potential side effects.

Did you always trust that the American Dental Association (ADA) and the Federal Drug Enforcement Agency (FDEA) would protect your health? Rest assured it wasn't easy for me to become disillusioned with dentists after listening to their opinions and advice while believing that it was their duty to protect my health and safety. I always believed I wouldn't want to lose my license after all those years of training either, but would I feel detrimental side effects of a material place in someone's body. I am positive that I would find a way to protect another human being without sacrificing my license or self. I expected that medical associations and governmental agencies were protecting our society.

If mercury is one of the most poisonous substances known to man, why did my dentist put it in my mouth? Mercury toxicity should be the lead poisoning of the twenty-first century.

5

What's the Difference?

Another term for silver fillings is *amalgam fillings*. This type of filling consists of metals—copper, silver, tin, zinc, and liquid mercury. When these metals are combined to create fillings, the largest portion is composed of mercury.

It seems that more dentists prefer the amalgam fillings because they are stronger, longer-lasting, and a less-expensive material.

When I visited the dentist for a reassessment of the dental work in my mouth due to my newfound awareness of the long-term toxic effects associated with silver fillings and other metals, he didn't seem concerned at all. My dentist stated that he has never had anyone complain that their fillings or crowns had affected their health in any way. I expressed to him that I felt most people wouldn't complain to their dentist about their general health or ailments but rather sores in their mouth or toothaches.

I find that when people are given a choice of dental fillings, they usually choose the amalgam fillings because of the price difference, not knowing that they are paying for *poison*.

The composite fillings are white in color and made up of a powder of ground glass mixed with a plastic binder. They require more time than amalgam fillings (silver) to harden. Also more expensive than amalgam fillings, the composite fillings are much more attractive than the amalgam fillings and are also *poison-free*. It seems that most dentists don't favor the composite fillings because they feel that they will only hold up for six years compared to amalgam fillings that will hold up for twelve or more. I'd rather get a filling that only holds up for six years and know that I am not being poisoned. My life is much more important than the life of my filling.

I learned that there are hundreds of different materials that can be used in the composite (white) fillings. Even though this filling is not poisonous, you could still be highly allergic to the material that is used in this type of filling.

You will soon learn how important the serum compatibility test is for wellness. This test will show you which composite materials (white fillings) you are *least reactive* to.

Questions

1. Would you go to a dentist to ask questions about your physical or mental health?
2. Did you know that *mercury* is in your amalgam (silver) fillings?
3. Did you ever think that a dentist would put *poisons* in your mouth or materials that you could be *allergic* to that could affect your immune system?

Mercury is a cytotoxin. It is poisonous to all living cells!

CYTOTOXIN

A substance (as a toxin or antibody) having a toxic effect on cells. *(Webster's Dictionary)*

6

Did You Ever Think the Mercury Used in Your Amalgam Fillings Could Make You Ill?

I don't need a doctor, scientist, or dentist to convince me that mercury, being a poison, could have an adverse effect upon my health.

When you have a hair mineral analysis test, the levels of metals found in your body, including mercury, are recorded. If the mercury level recorded is low, wouldn't you think that it could still have a significantly detrimental effect upon your health since any level of poison is harmful?

Who would want any level of mercury in their body, especially a person who is highly sensitive to this substance?

Dr. Huggins believes that it is not only the presence of mercury that counts, but also a person's *reaction* to it. A very small amount of mercury can be a serious problem for people who are highly allergic (sensitive) to it.

I not only had high levels of mercury but I was also highly allergic, which explains why I was dying.

The serum compatibility test will show you how allergic you are to various metals, including mercury.

TROUBLES ARE OFTEN THE TOOLS BY WHICH
GOD FASHIONS US FOR BETTER THINGS!

—H. W. Beecher

7

Mercury Toxicity and How It Affects Your Body

I asked myself, could it be possible for the mercury in my body to give me all these ailments, too many to count? Every day upon awakening, I would have another ailment. When I had all the metals in my mouth removed, the ailments started fading away overnight. Yes, it's true! Your symptoms could be much different than mine, as no two people are the same.

In the book *It's All in Your Head*, it states that this is one of the more difficult questions to answer because mercury attacks the body in so many ways. When mercury interferes with energy production and oxygen transport, all cells in the body are affected.

Mercury is the only heavy metal that causes a blockage in the conversion of body-formed chemicals called *porphyrins* into *hemoglobin* and the energy storage called *ATP.* Blocking this process is robbing your body of energy needed for repair and normal activity. This helps me understand where chronic fatigue comes in.

POLYPHYRINS

Any of various compounds containing four pyrrole rings, occurring universally in protoplasm, and functioning as a metal-binding cofactor in hemoglobin, chlorophyll, and certain enzymes. (American Heritage Dictionary)

ATP

An adenosine-derived nucleotide, $C_{10}H_{16}N_5O_{13}P_3$ that contains high energy phosphate bonds and is used to transport energy to cells for biochemical processes, including muscle contraction and enzymatic metabolism, though its hydrolysis to ADP. ATP is hydrolyzed to AMP when it is incorporated into DNA or RNA. (American Heritage Dictionary)

PROTOPLASM

The complex, semi fluid, translucent substance that constitutes the living matter of plant and animal cells and manifests the essential life functions of a cell. Composed of proteins, fats, and other molecules suspended in water, it includes the nucleus and cytoplasm. (American Heritage Dictionary)

HEMOGLOBIN

The iron containing respiratory pigment in red blood cells of vertebrates, consisting of about 6% heme and 94% globin. Hemoglobin's primary function is to transport oxygen from the lungs to all body tissues. (American Heritage Dictionary)

Heme

The deep red, non-protein, ferrous (iron) component of hemoglobin, $C_{34}H_{32}FeN_4O_4$. (American Heritage Dictionary)

Globin

The protein constituent of hemoglobin and myoglobin. (American Heritage Dictionary)

Myoglobin

A single chain, iron-containing protein found in muscle fibers, structurally similar to a single subunit of hemoglobin and having a higher affinity for oxygen than hemoglobin of the blood. (American Heritage Dictionary)

8

Alarming Information

The American Dental Association has been very reluctant to acknowledge that mercury amalgams (silver fillings) are toxic. Why are they hesitant to communicate with their members the recent alarming evidence that shows the role in physical illness that the mercury used in amalgams (silver fillings) can have? Mercury is considered a cytotoxin, and *Webster's-Dictionary* states that cytotoxins are poisonous substances. Would you want a poisonous substance in your body? The ADA feels that mercury amalgam fillings are safe because they don't vaporize or form toxic compounds to a significant degree when hardened.

As a result, I believe many dentists are unaware of the harm caused by mercury. Are most dentists ignorant of the substantial body of solid scientific research that already exists on mercury toxicity from dental fillings? Is it because scientists in fields other than dentistry have performed the majority of scientific studies and data?

I suppose that their teachers, professional associations, and colleagues have told the majority of dentists that amalgam fillings are safe as long as they harden. Please don't be surprised if your dentist tells you that silver fillings have positively no effect on your health because so many dentists gave me the same information.

During a dental visit, I told the dentist that I had read that some research showed that the mercury used in dental fillings have caused stomach and intestinal pain similar to the severe type that

I was experiencing. He told me that he had never heard of anyone having a problem such as mine. I was a little upset by this remark and told him that people probably would go to an internist or their family physician if they were having problems with their digestive system, never suspecting that silver fillings and other metals could be the culprits.

I recommend getting the serum compatibility test, which tests an individual's *sensitivity* to mercury and all other metals. Most dentists will not argue with a medical test and would replace any dental work with a compatible material immediately.

Procedures are followed in most dental offices every day, contradicting the irrational theory that mercury (silver fillings) is safe. Have you ever noticed that mercury fillings, which have been in your mouth for years, become treated as *toxic waste* the moment they are removed from your mouth? Dentists must place discarded fillings and extracted teeth containing mercury into hazardous waste receptacles for proper disposal. All of these waste receptacles are labeled as well, and notification is clearly made that these trash bins contain *hazardous* materials.

Isn't it ironic that the American Dental Association thinks that mercury-silver filings are completely safe and harmless when inside people's mouths for twenty-four hours every day, but when discarded, they become treated as *dangerous toxic waste* and are an *environmental hazard*?

Technology was very primitive when mercury amalgam was introduced into this country as a dental filling material in the year 1833. It wasn't possible to prove with scientific data that dentists shouldn't use the amalgams, which were inexpensive and long-lasting.

I feel that the American Dental Association hasn't taken full responsibility for our safety and health regarding dental care. It is for this reason that I want to share my newfound awareness—a shocking realization about the dangers of mercury and other potentially harmful metals used in the practice of dentistry.

TOXIC

1. Of, relating to, or caused by a toxin or other poison.
2. Capable of causing injury or death, especially by chemical means, poisonous. (*American Heritage Dictionary*)

POISON

1. A substance that causes injury, illness or death, especially by chemical means. Something destructive or fatal.
2. *Chemistry & Physics*—A substance that inhibits another substance or a reaction. (*American Heritage Dictionary*)

9

Scandalous News

It was so shocking to me when I found out that only a handful of practicing dentists are actually protecting our health.

I hope that it is because most dentists, men and women bearing good will, just don't know any better. Research, studies, and the collection of data are crucial to reach definitive conclusions concerning the detrimental effects of mercury on the public's health. It is so important to educate dental practitioners who support its use.

I hope that more and more conscientious dental professionals will soon become aware of the toxic effects of mercury (silver fillings) and other metals used in dentistry and join the rebellion against their use!

THE DIFFICULTIES WE EXPERIENCE ALWAYS
ILLUMINATE THE LESSONS WE NEED MOST!

—Unknown

10

My Journey to Wellness

In 1986, a year before my husband suffered a fatal heart attack, I started to have flu-like symptoms twenty-four hours a day. I woke up every morning thinking that these symptoms should surely be gone by now. However, I continuously had a sore throat, headaches, swollen glands, body aches and pains, unusual fatigue; and my tonsils were the size of golf balls.

After having these persistent flu-like symptoms for one month, I went to see a medical doctor. After examining my throat, he gave me a dose of antibiotics for two weeks, asking me to check back with him if I didn't feel any better after that time. He seemed sure that I would be just fine. Two weeks later, I returned to his office with the same symptoms with absolutely no change. During this visit, he prescribed a two-week course of Amoxicillin, a broad-spectrum antibiotic. By the time the second treatment of antibiotics was finished, I felt as though my condition was worse.

Almost imperceptibly, my strength began slipping away. Upon awakening, I would lie in bed with tears running down my cheeks while trying to figure out how I would find the strength to get through the day to tend to the needs of my three beautiful children ages three, five, and seven years. It was so very frightening!

I returned a third time for a visit with my physician. He advised me that there wasn't anything else that he could do and referred me to an ear, nose, and throat specialist.

During this visit, the doctor highly recommended that I have my tonsils removed. Desperately trusting this physician with my health and all my heart, I took his advice and checked into the hospital a week later to have my tonsils removed.

I couldn't wait until the operation was over. Feeling extremely excited, I now believed that I would be so much better after the surgery. Just to know that the doctor actually promised that I would start to see my symptoms disappear shortly after the removal of my tonsils was encouraging. The recovery was painful and long. However, *after the surgery*, I was devastated when I realized that the only thing that disappeared were my tonsils. The rest of the symptoms continued as full-blown maladies while I developed new ones every day.

Overnight, my stomach became sensitive to certain foods. My thinking was foggy, and I was confused all of the time. The fatigue continued and even increased as I struggled to make it through a day. In the evening, I would collapse into bed, not having enough strength or energy to change into my sleepwear.

My outside appearance looked just fine. My husband and friends took my lethargy (which was caused by my health issues), personally, thinking that I had a disinterested attitude. Losing my friends was a painful experience. I felt so alone. I would not dare tell anyone that I developed new and more distressing symptoms every day for fear that they would think that I was going insane. I made up excuses for myself to cover my illness.

Since I didn't have enough strength to be sexually active with my husband, he started to accuse me of having an affair with another man. I would silently cry as I desperately wished that he could understand for just one second how weak I felt.

I was even too weak to fight for the truth. My husband continued to be angry as he questioned whether I was really sick or making this all up. He insisted that I find a new doctor. I had no clue where to turn next, as I cried all day after he would leave for work. While wondering why everyone was punishing me for feeling sick, I became increasingly frightened about my health.

Following my husband's wishes, I went to see a different medical doctor who didn't think that this was very serious or anything to be alarmed about. He diagnosed me as severely depressed and believed that a vacation would do me wonders. Crying, I tried to convince the doctor that I really had nothing to be depressed about; my only depression would be me feeling so ill and scared that no doctor or testing was giving me any answers. Being very confused and frustrated during the consultation with this doctor, I asked him why the glands in my neck were swollen and painful? He told me that depression could do a lot of damage to a person's body. Of course, the doctor's answers were not what I was looking for.

My husband desperately wanted me to return to the way I used to be. He took the doctor's recommendation and booked a trip to the Caribbean for seven days. He was still upset with me, as he felt that I was not very excited or appreciative about taking this extravagant vacation. I could not help but be more frightened than excited about this trip because I had no strength. Just the thought of pacing a suitcase wore me out. My husband hired someone to help me prepare for the trip since he always did try his best to please me.

We went on the trip, and I worried every day that something was going to happen to me health-wise. The flu-like symptoms continued, and all I really wanted was to stay in bed all day. I didn't take part in any extra activities except to lounge on the beach all day. I don't know if it was my imagination, but *lying in the sun made my symptoms worse.*

After returning home from the trip, I was more depressed than ever. Inside my heart, I kept repeating, "God, what is wrong with me? Please help me!" The vacation certainly did not make a difference for me at all. While being so extremely fatigued, I continued to hold on for dear life, always having the fear of whether I could make it to the next day.

My family lived three hundred miles away and had no idea what was going on with my health. I knew that my mother would worry herself sick if I told her the truth, so I would just mention that I was very fatigued and could not understand the reason. She told me that she would be tired, too, if she had three little ones to take care of. I gave her statement serious thought, but I knew in my heart that I was overwhelmed by a totally different kind of tiredness. No matter how much I slept, I could not recover any energy. I was even afraid to climb stairs, attributing my uncanny exhaustion to a weak heart. I continued to keep my health problems a secret most of the time, as I feared that everyone would think that I was losing my mind since all the physicians that I visited couldn't find anything wrong with me.

Unexpectedly, two weeks after the trip, my husband collapsed and died right in front of me. He was only forty-two years old. The ambulance transporting him to the hospital pronounced him dead and attributed the cause to a massive heart attack with no known reason. I was in a state of shock. My husband had never complained or had any heart trouble or alarming symptoms, nor was he ever sick during our marriage.

I was now feeling that my symptoms were definitely a warning sign that something was seriously wrong with me. Could our home or drinking water be poisoning me? I couldn't understand why my world and health seemed to just crumble within months, becoming a total nightmare.

Desperately wanting to run away from everything and believing that our home was possibly the cause, I decided six months after my husband's death to hire a mover so that my children and I could live in the beach house that we owned two hours away on the Jersey shore. My love for the ocean made me long for its smell and sounds. The move proved to be too much for me, and I wound up in the hospital with severe dehydration and diarrhea for two weeks. Being sick and alone in an area where I was not established and didn't even know my neighbors made my life more complicated and difficult.

My brother flew down for a vacation from our hometown in Rochester, New York, while I was hospitalized. My father was dying with cancer at this time. I can remember my brother telling me that I looked worse than my father who was on his deathbed. Fortunately, my brother was able to help with my children. I was no longer able to hide my illness from my family.

During my stay at the hospital, my symptoms continued and at a higher level. The doctors continuously ordered every painful test possible. After seven days, all tests came back negative. The doctors informed me that there wasn't anything wrong with me except habitual and severe depression.

They recommended medication. I refused to take the medication prescribed for depression; and the doctors became enraged, dismissing my complaints, releasing me from the hospital, and labeling me a malingerer. I felt as though they were just sending me home to die. Discouraged with these doctors, since all they wanted to do was drug me, I came to despise all of them.

11

Herbal Potions

Now I needed full-time, live-in help. My nanny was named Sally. She was doing everything for me, even helping me take a shower. After showering, I would need to lie down before I could dry myself off because I felt like my heart would stop if I didn't.

Being bedridden most of the time and more desperate than ever to find a cure, I learned of a holistic practitioner who treated his patients with herbs. After his secretary explained the program to me, I became incredibly hopeful and excited and booked an appointment. During my visit, the doctor explained that my body was surmounted with toxins and that they had accumulated over many years. I felt like I had been poisoned and agreed with him. It made so much sense to me, but I couldn't understand where these awful toxins could be coming from, and the doctor didn't have a clue either. I bought hundreds of dollars of supplements for detoxifying my body. He was totally confident that I would feel wonderful in three months, and I was ecstatic!

Shortly after arriving home, I started the herbal treatment. Two days later, I was put in the hospital again with severe diarrhea, dehydration, and extreme dizziness. I felt that my body was detoxifying too fast. I showed the doctors the herbal remedies that I had been taking. They told me that these herbs were nothing but garbage and forbid me from taking them again. Being as so many people believed that holistic practitioners are scam artists, I kept my visits a secret.

No one was supportive, and I felt so alone. A dear friend who lived thousands of miles away phoned me a couple times a week, wishing that she lived close. She showed me tons of support. I was so confused. The holistic doctor was the first to make so much sense and give me any constructive advice although I couldn't understand why the treatments had made me feel so much sicker.

I didn't know anything about detoxification (cleansing the body of toxins). I prayed to find the right treatment and felt like I was coming closer to the solution every day. No matter how weak, fatigued, or bothered by brain fog, I was still determined to find the cure and become healthy again. I knew that I had to take charge. I imagined that everyone had given up on me and thought that I wanted to die.

I desperately continued searching for the answer. I needed to be there for my children. My dream had always been to be a mother and play a major part in their lives. They loved me so much, making my life complete. I tried to keep my daily focus on what I still had to be thankful for. Of course, my children were at the very top of my list. The worst thing that I could have imagined would be blindness from my illness and not being capable of seeing my three beautiful children's loving faces again.

12

Is Nutrition the Key?

I was now introduced to a lady that was totally devoted to the benefits of juicing using fresh fruits and vegetables. She came to my home and was quite thrilled to help, believing that juicing would facilitate my journey to find ways to become healthy once again. She mentioned that I was probably detoxifying much too fast for my system when I took the herbal medicine and introduced me to a book called *Juicing for Life* by Cherie Calbom that had saved her life. I purchased an expensive juicer, believing that using only organic vegetables and fruits would save my life. I *know* that fresh fruits and vegetables are the richest food source available and provide vitamins, minerals, and enzymes. The fresh juice tasted great, but my *stomach and intestines were raw, bloated, and unable to handle them,* putting an end to the juicing. I felt like my insides were overtaken with sores even though I had been eating very bland food. I had to put the juicer to rest in the closet.

I FEARED PAIN UNTIL I REALIZED THAT IT IS NECESSARY FOR GROWTH!
—Unknown

13

Could Allergies Be a Cause?

I was now experiencing much higher levels of anxiety, emotional instability, and awakening in the middle of the night. I also found myself sweating profusely and feeling totally confused. Numerous aches and pains, continual weight loss, severe phobias, an excessive metallic taste in my mouth, severe depression, and constant diarrhea plagued me too. The diarrhea was so serious that I had to be rushed to the emergency room four times in one month due to severe dehydration and pain. Even though I would drink at least eight glasses of water daily, the cause of the dehydration was still a mystery. There wasn't any medication that would make a difference either. Whenever I ate something sweet or with caffeine, all my disturbing symptoms intensified.

I soon followed a totally healthy diet plan without any soda, caffeine, or junk food—all to no avail. The purchase of an expensive reverse osmosis system for the house to purify the drinking water made no difference either.

I soon started to go to a chiropractor twice a week for the pain in my lower back and neck. The treatment helped the pain for a while, but it didn't last. If I didn't continue treatments on a regular basis, I would suffer with migraines and excruciating pain in my lower back.

I read an article about how food allergies could affect the body, causing many of my symptoms, so I invested in a series of food allergy tests. The results showed that I was highly reactive to dairy, wheat, eggs, and soy. I stopped eating these foods and totally substituted them with other foods, but still there was no change for the better.

14

Prescription for Addiction

Months went by, and I was still bedridden, unable to drive, and too fatigued to take a shower alone. My troubling symptoms continued to become increasingly worse, and I was forced to seek the advice of yet another medical doctor out of panic and fear. Upon my visits, the doctor stepped into the room to ask me the same questions that I had been asked before. Becoming so annoyed at trying to explain these same symptoms over and over again, I felt the need to write them all down and make copies so I could just hand them out as I went along from doctor to doctor. Though I was an obedient and good patient, I felt like this was a waste of my time and money once again.

Starting to cry, I explained my newest symptom to the doctor—of how I felt as if my lungs and brain were bleeding internally. The consultation was intensive, and he came to believe that I was extremely depressed and stressed due to the sudden loss of my beloved husband. I told him that I was too sick to even think about him. He insisted that I was extremely traumatized from my husband's sudden death and that I was having a hard time getting over such a terrifying experience.

I tried to explain that all my challenging symptoms began before my husband's death, but he ignored me. He prescribed Xanax instead to make me feel better, help me relax, and conquer my depression. Knowing that I would become dependent on this drug to alleviate my depression, I still asked him if it was addictive. He made me feel really stupid, covering up the intensely addictive nature of this drug.

I was never a believer in psychotropic or any type of prescription drugs, but I remember that the last time I had been hospitalized, they wanted me to take something for my depression. I listened to this doctor even though my heart was telling me otherwise. I knew that I was neither a medical doctor nor did I have a degree. I was raised to believe that a doctor is God, and if he prescribes medication, then you should take it without question because the doctor is never wrong.

I had the prescription filled and started to take the Xanax. Even though I didn't like the way it made me feel, I kept taking them for two weeks before returning to the doctor. At this time, I explained that I didn't like the way that this medicine made me feel, but he assured me that it would take some time for my body to adjust to it. Crying as I told him that my symptoms were totally impervious to this medication, I stressed how I slept all day and felt extremely confused. All the doctor did was ask me to have patience and continue to take the Xanax.

One evening, after three weeks of using Xanax, my daughter came into my room in the middle of the night crying in fear, trying her hardest to wake me up for help, without any luck. The next morning, I was shocked to hear that our dog, barking and growling profusely while in his cage in the living room, had awakened Shanna. I could hear the terror in her voice as she relived the horrifying experience and told me that she could not wake me.

A few hours later, I realized that all my uninsured and expensive jewelry had been stolen. These thieves could have killed me in my sleep and then proceeded to murder my children. We would have never had a chance if they were murderers.

I now believed that the devil was standing over me at all times. I started burning sage after being told that it would keep evil away. Until I had started taking Xanax, I had always been a light sleeper, but now fear ripped through me as I realized that this medication was putting me into a coma at night. I decided to take half of the prescribed dose, which made a difference. After this experience, I doubted that a doctor could really know the strength or type of medication that was right for another individual or how it would affect them.

I WILL APPRECIATE THAT ALL OF MY INSTINCTS AND FEELINGS EXIST FOR A REASON. TODAY, INSTEAD OF TRYING TO BANISH THESE FEELINGS, I WILL STRIVE TO FIND A BALANCE.

—Unknown

15

Suspicion of AIDS

A few days after the robbery of our home and the loss of my jewelry, I purchased a magazine with a detailed and lengthy article about AIDS. I started reading but shortly put the magazine down in a panic, as I realized that every symptom described here matched mine. Afraid to continue reading, I called my doctor and requested that another AIDS test be done, thinking that they have misdiagnosed the last test. I remember being in such a panic, as well as being somewhat relieved, to feel that at least I would now know what was wrong with me.

When I went into the doctor's office to have the test repeated, he demanded that I admit myself into the hospital immediately. Drowning in my own tears and frightened, I went even though I knew how dreadful and painful the tests to be repeated on me would be. After a two-week stay in the hospital, I had every possible test. I started sobbing as the doctor read me the results for all of the tests. They had come back negative, and through the process of elimination, he was sure that it was just my nerves. I now felt that I surely must be crazy.

The doctor suggested that a vacation would do me a world of good and help me get away from all of my upsetting memories. Could he be right when I knew in my heart that a vacation was not the answer, but only a means of escape from a mysterious illness that was ruining my life. I was more perplexed and baffled than before because now I felt as though I was definitely losing my mind. Who was I to argue with the doctor convinced that I was just a crazy lady? If it were not for the love of my children, I would have certainly taken my life.

After returning from the hospital, I was still bedridden, quite scared, and more discouraged than ever. I almost gave up my struggle for survival, but after two months, I began searching for the answers and fought to regain my health. I kept wondering if the much-advised vacation was really possible for I hardly had enough strength to go to the bathroom. I decide to discuss this with my live-in nanny, Sally, to see what she would suggest. She told me that if I thought that this would help, she would be there for me and do whatever possible to make this vacation happen. She even promised to help me secure a wheelchair and arrange the entire trip. She assured me that she would be more than happy to help my children and me by coming with us on our vacation.

She made the reservations for the week of Easter vacation, when the five of us would fly to Marco Island, Florida. Being extremely fatigued on the vacation, I could only sit on the porch of our condo and watch my children swim. The rest of the time, I was bedridden and worried again about whether I could gather up the strength for the flight home on the plane.

I was awakened on Friday morning with dizziness, unbearable body and joint pain, extreme nausea, trouble breathing, and body tremors that I had no control over. My live-in nanny wasn't sure where the hospital was but felt that I needed to get to one immediately. She saw a gentleman standing outside our condo and decided to ask him for help. This man informed us that there wasn't a hospital on Marco Island, but he did know of an excellent medical doctor on the island. This man called a cab, and we arrived in five minutes.

The good doctor took me in as an emergency. After taking one look at me, he told me that I was not only dehydrated but extremely toxic, as well. This was the first time that I had ever heard that I was toxic from a medical doctor. Wasting no time, he hooked me up to a multivitamin intravenous solution and started to pose a few questions to me, when I suddenly started to cry and asked him if I was going to die. He comforted and reassured me by taking my hand and saying, "Donna, if you stick with me, you won't die."

I told him that every doctor had thought I was a malingering lunatic that just wanted attention, but he challenged his diagnosis by telling me that my symptoms were very much real. He knew that the yellow color on the bottom of my feet and the palms of my hands were significant physical attributes caused by a liver that was being overloaded with toxins. I could see that he wanted to help me as he continued to ask me questions in order to figure out how I had become so toxic, but I had no idea how this could have happened to me.

At that moment, I felt so blessed to have met this physician because I could see that he was aware of my toxic appearance, something quite obvious, that no other doctor had ever recognized. The doctor told me that he would administer multivitamin intravenous solutions that would help remove the toxins from my body. When the doctor saw that I had finished the intravenous drip, he told me to return to his office the next morning. He obliged me to call the office's phone service if I had any problems before then. This doctor could not have had any idea of the comfort and hope that he had given me. Though I felt very sick throughout the night, I was able to remain stable until morning.

I was back at the doctor's office the following morning to receive another multivitamin intravenous solution. I was elated to have finally found a supportive medical doctor. Only one day was left before we were to depart for our return trip to New Jersey, but I knew that I needed to stay on the island and continue to receive the treatments that the doctor had begun. This was the first treatment that I had received since my illness began other than the prescription of Xanax, a drug used to just mask my illness but to never cure it.

I felt so stressed as I was forced to tell my children that they would be going home with the nanny while I remained on Marco Island to continue with the treatments. I am sure that my poor little children wondered if they would ever see their mother again. I tried to reassure them that I needed to remain in Florida in order to become well so that we could be a happy, healthy, and active family. My heart ached as they departed on their flight back home to New

Jersey. It was ever so hard, as I worried about them every day, waiting for their phone call, only to hear them cry for me to return home.

I continued with the intravenous multivitamin treatments for five days a week for one month. I was so lonely as I didn't know a soul in Florida. I was somewhat afraid of being alone at night in the event that I would become so ill that I couldn't get up to use the telephone for help. Fortunately, this never happened. These special intravenous treatments were stabilizing my health and keeping me out of the hospital, which was very encouraging.

The testing continued during this time. When the results came back, the doctor told me that I had a severely abnormal white blood cell and red blood cell count *that couldn't be identified with any known disease.* It was at this time that the doctor told me that I had the worst case of chronic fatigue syndrome he had ever seen as all my symptoms were the only markers for this mysterious illness.

The doctor was in total shock when I told him that no physician had ever mentioned or diagnosed this condition. Ironically, I was happy to know that I now had a real disease with a real name finally convincing me that I wasn't crazy. In his next breath, the doctor told me that the medical field had no known cure for chronic fatigue syndrome at this time. Of course, my optimism turned to despair as I now considered that I might just feel like this for the rest of my life.

The doctor could see that I was despondent. He then explained his theory about the treatments that he used to help his patients feel better, as they learned to cope with the devastating illness of chronic fatigue. He believed that the multivitamin intravenous solution he administered would help to strengthen the immune system and cleanse the toxins from my body. Stress reduction exercises were also used and thought to be very beneficial. I now attempted Tai Chi, medication, and walking. I only could cope with the meditation.

At the end of the four weeks of treatment, I felt a little stronger. I now knew that I could at least remain stable and sit up in my seat for the plane trip home. I had no idea what I was thinking, but I just wanted to get home to my children. I certainly wasn't thinking of myself, feeling as though I was so distanced from them. I told the doctor that I needed to get back to New Jersey to be with my children, and he wished me well. The next day I was on the plane to go home, but as I arrived, fear came over me all of a sudden. I hadn't thought about it before, but now I wondered what I would do if the attacks returned or my health started to decline again.

Sure enough, two days after I arrived home to New Jersey, I was rushed to the hospital with severe dehydration and diarrhea and forced to stay and endure more testing. I was so sick again that as I stood up, my body started to shake with miserable tremors. In the hospital, I explained to the doctor that I had been diagnosed with chronic fatigue syndrome while visiting Florida. I also told him about the treatments they had used to help stabilize the progression of this malady. However, he just seemed to ignore me as he told me that he had never heard of any such remedies. I felt like this doctor wasn't interested in the bewildering disease of chronic fatigue syndrome, or did he care about the treatments that were helping me either. The painful tests began again; even an agonizing spinal tap was executed.

Several different medications were also prescribed. I didn't want them because they were making me feel even sicker, but I was too weak to fight their orders and afraid to refuse the doctors' advice. I could only pray for God's help to somehow get me back to Florida; for if I couldn't go, I felt as though I would surely die.

Three days later, I knew that I needed to find the strength to sign myself out of this hospital. I finally found the strength to call my nanny and see if she could book a flight to Florida as soon as possible. As I spoke, my heart felt like it would just quit beating, for just a simple phone call was too much work for me.

The nanny arranged the flight for the next day. She also contacted a Realtor who knew of a furnished home that we could rent only three miles away from the Marco Island doctor's office. A rental car and a household assistant to stay with us on Marco Island were also arranged. The assistant would have to do everything, including all the driving, shopping, cooking, cleaning, and even take care of my children. I signed myself out of the hospital that evening as the nurses stared at me as if I was crazy. I guess that I wasn't that crazy because I am still alive today.

My children and I went to the airport the next morning. When we arrived in Florida, they pushed me in a wheelchair through the airport since I was too weak to walk. *Everything was perfect* when we arrived in Florida. The hired help had everything ready, even a home-made dinner, when we got to our rented home on Marco Island. I phoned the doctor that evening and left a message with his phone service desperately explaining how important it was for the doctor to return my call. He returned my phone call immediately and met me at his office that evening. I added how sick I had become after arriving in New Jersey, only to wind up in the hospital once again.

I was given an intravenous of the multivitamin solution. Tearfully, I told the doctor that I was so ecstatic to be back in Florida and that I thought I was going to die while in the hospital in New Jersey. I was too sick to care that I had to leave my beach home, dog, horse, and other treasured belongings behind. I finally had to face that I had to give nearly everything I owned away since my illness left me too incapacitated to worry about proper storage or care for these important things in my life. I couldn't worry about pets or material things. I had no other choice at this point in time, as I was fighting to save my life.

I continued receiving the treatments of the multivitamin solution intravenously five days a week for three months until the doctor went on a two-week vacation. I knew that these treatments were keeping me out of the hospital and helping me make progress since I was able to sit up for much longer periods of time, and my stomach was feeling a little better and was now able to introduce more foods into my diet.

16

A Long Journey to Nowhere

While the good doctor was on vacation, I was not receiving any treatments, and I could feel myself slipping backward. I felt that I would need these IV treatments for the rest of my life. During the doctor's absence, a friend from New Jersey called and told me how she had known someone with chronic fatigue syndrome, who went to a detoxification center in Los Angeles, feeling 70 percent better after the completion of the program she was enrolled in. This sounded like the perfect solution to me, a detoxification center helping those afflicted with chronic fatigue syndrome. This treatment center seemed so important to me since I never thought that I would ever feel 70 percent better again. I called the detoxification center and reserved a place in the program for the next week.

I felt that I needed this treatment desperately. My children's hearts were broken once again, as they were informed that they had to remain in Florida, while I went alone to Los Angeles for a new type of treatment. They were quite upset since they really had been in Florida for only three months and hadn't had much time to make new friends after leaving and missing all of their old ones in New Jersey. I explained how very important these treatments were to me and that I didn't want to continuously keep getting the IVs for the rest of my life.

Since I hadn't been getting the intravenous drips, I was experiencing severe body pain again. My lungs and brain felt like they were bleeding. I had blurred vision all of the time. I also had extreme brain fog, severe fatigue, regular diarrhea, and I was becoming severely depressed again. Feeling desperate again, I was rather excited about my flight to Los Angeles to try yet another cure for my chronic fatigue syndrome.

All I can remember about my six-hour flight to Los Angeles was that I was so very sick and fatigued that I didn't care if the plane crashed.

When I arrived at the Los Angeles airport, a driver, sent by the program, was waiting to take me to the hotel. He grabbed my luggage, and we were on our way. The area that the hotel was located in was a little scary looking to me, definitely not a first or even second-class hotel. I cried the whole night through, wanting to be back in Florida. I felt as though I was risking my life, just to save it, while staying in this frightening area. The next morning, I called a taxi to take me to the treatment center even though it was within walking distance because I didn't feel safe there, and I was also far too weak to walk just the one block to the center.

The nurses at the treatment center had no idea how hard it was for me to find the strength to answer their questions, as they filled out the paperwork during the check-in procedure. I could tell that the first doctor that examined me was a little shocked to see how sick I appeared. He informed me that I had to stop taking Xanax medication before I could begin the treatment plan. I started to cry as I told him how dependent I had become to this medication and that it would take at least two weeks for me to stop using it completely.

I felt so alone and confused with this insensitive man. Why didn't he ask me what medications I had been taking before signing me up for the program and asking me to travel so far away for their detoxification program and treatment plan?

I decided to tell the doctor about the trouble that I had with dehydration and how I had to be admitted to the hospital on several occasions due to this problem. The doctor told me that he wanted me to come to the clinic every day for intravenous solutions to prevent the dehydration. Now stuck in a seedy hotel room by myself for two weeks, too weak to go anywhere except to the clinic for my daily

IVs, I agonizingly quit my serious addiction to Xanax. The whole scenario was quite frightening, and I cried daily as I was at my lowest point and felt totally miserable.

I didn't trust any of the employees at the program after learning from one of the patients that it was run by scientologists. I was a little relieved that the doctor had at least ordered the daily intravenous solutions to keep me from dehydrating. I was too ashamed to share my thoughts of impending doom or my fear of dying out in Los Angeles, completely alone.

My children called me on the telephone every day, crying and begging for me to come home. My life felt as though it was being sucked out of me. The program was costing me thousands upon thousands of dollars. I was also paying a hundred dollar daily for the hotel, which was a high-priced dump.

I FEARED PAIN UNTIL I LEARNED THAT IT IS NECESSARY FOR GROWTH!
—Unknown

17

A Seed Is Planted

After a two-week period of time, I was able to stop using the Xanax completely. Although this was quite a struggle for me, I was finally ready and looking forward to begin the treatments. When I went to check in to the clinic and given a pre-physical for the program, they told me that I was much too sick to endure their detoxification program.

Instead of letting me use the detoxification program that I had paid for, they invited me to come to the clinic every day to sit in the sauna, which was a safer method of detoxifying my body. I really believed this offer was just a tactic to justify keeping the thousands of dollars that I had given them for the program, but I was too sick to argue or fight for what I felt was right. I was so desperate for a cure that I would try any treatment recommended.

After a month of the sauna treatments, which were absolutely useless, I knew that I had to get back to Florida. Sicker and more confused than ever before, my brain fog had increased, and I was petrified of flying back to Florida alone. I decided to ask a gentleman in the program, whom I had become friendly with, named Richard, if he would escort me back to Florida. I was afraid to venture home by myself, alone and unaided. I even offered to buy him a round-trip ticket if he would do this immense favor for me. He could see how sick I was and empathized with my dilemma as he had just been cured of cancer. Richard was happy to accompany me home and be of help.

I was dizzy most of the time, and my vision was so blurred that I couldn't read any signs on the way to the airport. I felt like the walking dead as we boarded the plane, knowing that nobody could imagine how much I dreaded this flight. I felt like crawling into a corner to die, but the thought of seeing my children soon kept me from doing that. We made it back to Florida, and Richard promised to keep in touch after his return to California.

About two months after Richard had returned to California, he called to tell me that he had just finished reading an important article and sounded very excited. He told me that he now knew what was making me so sick. I asked him what he wanted me to do, thinking that he was going to give me another miracle cure to try. He started reading the article to me over the phone. It was about silver fillings and the serious reactions that some people have to them. He seemed so sure that the gray fillings that he had seen in my teeth were the cause of the problems that I was having with my health.

I thought that this assumption was outrageous. There was nothing wrong with my teeth. I had just spent a fortune on them. A qualified dentist, who was also a member of the ADA performed numerous procedures including porcelain crowns, fillings, and root canals to give me a beautiful smile. I was sure that he would never put anything harmful into my mouth. This whole idea seemed crazy to me, and I told him that I wasn't going to fall for this gimmick. We continued to debate this issue for a while when I finally said that the American Dental Association would never allow dentists to continue using any materials that were harmful. As far as I was concerned, the case was closed, and the topic was never mentioned again. We remained friends!

I FEARED CHANGE UNTIL I SAW THAT EVEN TO THE
MOST BEAUTIFUL BUTTERFLY HAD TO UNDERGO A
METAMORPHOSIS BEFORE IT COULD FLY!

—Unknown

18

Not the Only One

Once again, I started to receive the intravenous multivitamin drip, at least twice a week from the Marco Island doctor. This was the only treatment that kept me stable and helped to remove a lot of the aches and pains throughout my body. Without a doubt, this treatment was helpful, but progress was slower than I had expected. About halfway through the treatment, my veins already weakened from the toxins, would collapse, and the needle would have to be reinserted into a new vein. After a while, there were no more areas in my arms to insert the needles, so they had to be injected into the top of my foot. This didn't burn as much and seemed to work a great deal better, which was somewhat of an improvement.

I soon started attending the group that the doctor had sponsored for those who suffered from chronic fatigue syndrome. There were six females in this support group. We were extremely desperate, suffering with similar symptoms, but most importantly, we were all extremely fatigued. Meeting others, who had no idea where to turn for help, gave me the feeling that I wasn't alone with this dreadful illness.

We all felt like the doctor on Marco Island was the only physician who cared or understood our needs. Since we didn't have any broken bones, looked fine on the outside, and were not in need of any surgery, most people were baffled by our illness. We all felt that we were definitely fortunate to be under the tutelage of this good doctor, who wanted to understand our affliction and help cure us from this disabling illness.

The multivitamin intravenous drops were continued for at least six months, twice a week. I started to regain some of my strength. Now I was able to go for car rides and shower myself without having to lay down to rest before being able to dry myself off. This was encouraging, but I could tell that I still had a long road ahead.

After six months passed, a tooth bothered me. I avoided going to a dentist and used Advil for the pain instead. Once again, I couldn't believe that this was happening to me now. I couldn't imagine where I was going to find the strength to sit in a dentist's chair. I could remember the depression and not being able to get out of bed for at least a week when I last visited a dentist. This upsetting memory kept me from wanting to tend to the needs of my teeth. Although, I always mentioned these disabling aftereffects to the dentist, his lack of concern was frustrating, and as I reclined back into the dental chair, I always felt as though I was talking to the ceiling.

One morning upon awakening, my tooth was throbbing so much that I now realized that I had no choice but to seek the help of a dentist who set an appointment for me as soon as I called. After taking x-rays, the dentist informed me that the tooth would have to be pulled as it was beyond the point of being saved. He also wanted to perform a root canal on the adjacent tooth, as it was also decayed. I was so fatigued at this time that I could not imagine enduring a root canal procedure, so I had both of the teeth pulled. When he set the two extracted teeth on the tray in front, I couldn't help but notice the ugly gray color of the silver filling covering them. The dentist insisted that I return immediately for a cleaning, which I did. After the cleaning appointment, I was bedridden for weeks.

I was now totally confused. Why was my progress going backward? Instead of feeling better after having the much-needed dental work, I was sicker. My symptoms were so serious again that I had to receive three multivitamin IVs each week. I couldn't figure out why I felt as though I was being poisoned again. Discouraged again, my life was unbearable and dismal due to my illness.

My agonizing symptoms were full-blown again. I couldn't even go for a car ride because I was so weak. I was also plagued by unbelievable body pain, tremors, and a burning sensation inside the top of my head and inside my lungs. My fatigue escalated, and my goal of restored energy and vitality seemed impossible. My only activity was to travel from my bed to the doctor's office to receive the intravenous treatments. These were continued over a period of at least five months, three times a week.

During every IV treatment, the pain was so horrendous that I strained to hold back the tears. When I mentioned this to the doctor, he believed that the pain in my veins was caused by the toxicity. I couldn't comprehend this turmoil. I felt as though I had just begun to reach the top of a steep mountain, only to be sent back to the bottom overnight. I often wondered what I was doing to my body to deserve this torment.

I could only keep searching for the answers, for my goals had changed, and I was determined to never give up. Three months later, I started to feel better again. This encouraged me to remain positive and seek the solution.

I was now optimistic that I was on the path to recovery because at least driving short distances was possible. I can remember driving my children to sports activities, although I was still too weak to get out of the car to watch them play. I would rest in the back seat of the car so that I could conserve my strength to drive them back home.

Though somewhat improved, a daily nap was essential, and housework was out of the question. My children were now relieved and joyful. The minimal attention that I gave them seemed like a lot.

Every day, frequent periods of rest were necessary because overexertion would place me back in bed for weeks. At this time, the multivitamin treatments were administered once a week, which was quite an improvement.

I started seeing a holistic doctor who provided different natural herbal supplements to help give me more strength. He also prescribed natural enzymes to stabilize the flora in my stomach and natural remedies to help heal the sores covering the lining of my stomach and intestines. I considered these natural treatments because they were less painful than the intravenous solutions previously prescribed. I tried these remedies faithfully, but they only caused more pain in my stomach and intestinal area. At this point, the only thing I could drink was purified water.

I continued to see this holistic doctor for at least eight months, trying every treatment that he could offer, hoping that this was the answer. Colonics, Reiki, deep-tissue massage, aromatherapy, reflexology, hypnotism, magnetic bracelets, religion and prayer, manual lymph drainage, BodyTalk, acupuncture, meditation, and visualization were some of the therapies that were recommended and tried. Even though I tried them all, they were a waste of time and money. The only successful method that helped was the multivitamin treatment from the good doctor.

I would have my setbacks, but overall, I was doing much better. I was able to start doing things and going places that no longer gave me anxiety. Once in a while, my symptoms would start to kick in again, and I would get ever so scared. I still had to be so careful of what I ate as most foods still caused pain in my stomach and intestinal area. Yes, some days would still leave me quite sick; however, this was a huge improvement from my previous condition.

> WHEN WE BRING THINGS OUT INTO THE LIGHT,
> THEY LOSE THEIR POWER OVER US.
>
> —Anonymous

19

Self-Healing?

I had been attending weekly sessions with a chiropractor to help with the migraines and pains in my back and neck. This chiropractor knew how long I had been sick and that I was still struggling. He told me about a counselor that taught the art of self-healing and had even written a book on the subject. The chiropractor thought that I would be very interested since I appeared to be open-minded and would try anything to get well.

With much hesitation, I called and spoke to the secretary since I had tried so many remedies with no success. Still being dissatisfied with the condition of my health, I decided to give self-healing a try. Since there was a two-week wait for an appointment, I decided to purchase her book, *The Heroic Path*. Not knowing what to expect during the session, I was very nervous but feeling so grateful that I could still afford the extravagance of this visit. The woman, so loving and understanding, had experienced so much pain in her life, that I was further encouraged. She had experienced breast cancer twice but never lost her faith in God, thus giving her the courage to heal herself. I admired her bravery and faith so much. The self-healing therapy kept me mentally strong. I now believed that I was the only one that could find the answers to a cure that would save my life.

I found that the self-healing therapy helped me in so many ways. Not only did I feel empowered by her counseling, but it also helped me overcome the low self-esteem caused from the trauma and difficulties of my past, which, I felt at this time, could have possibly contributed to the chronic fatigue syndrome. Learning to love myself and trust God was pivotal in giving me the authority to now be responsible for my health and feel worthy of it.

After one-and-a-half years of attending the weekly sessions that instructed me on the art of self-healing, I still did not feel totally well and knew that something regarding my health and energy level was still not normal. Struggling to function and do normal daily activities, my frustration level remained high.

During my visit, I confided to the counselor that I was concerned about my health. I could not understand why I felt so ill after receiving dental work the week before. I told her that he had replaced a filling and a crown. Increased levels of depression, anxiety, daily migraines, and severe body pain troubled me afterward. My eyes remained red and swollen, as I spent much of the time crying in tears. I confronted her with my concerns about the problems now opposing my health. I wondered if the injection of Novocain had caused an allergic reaction or if the dentist could be the culprit of my illness.

Totally discouraged with her answers refuting my idea that the dental visits had contributed to my illness, I believed it was time to move on knowing that her self-healing methods could not provide the definitive or total solution to cure me of chronic fatigue syndrome. Discouragement not only forced me to stop seeing the counselor but also believe that chronic fatigue syndrome was something that I would have to learn to accept and live with forever.

Although self-healing was not the total answer to my illness, I achieved an abundance of inner strength and spirituality. What a wonderful tool this was, for it led me to trust and follow my dreams. Believing in something is the key to making it real. Knowing that dreams reveal so much about the inner self, I knew that I had to totally believe in them for them to become a reality.

While resting in my bed, my dreams were the center of my attention, revealing what I wanted to achieve in the future. My first dream was of becoming healthy, active, joyful, and pain-free. My second vision led me to my very own charming, modest, peach-colored cottage with classically elegant French doors on all sides. A white picket fence covered with flowering vines appeared, following the complete perimeter of the yard. Under a tall cypress shade tree, a radiant red-haired woman appeared, peacefully reading a book while sitting on an Adirondack chair, in a beautiful garden with blissfully chirping birds and striking butterflies flying around vibrant flowers. A large pedestal-style stone birdbath was nearby. Feeling strong enough mentally, my dreams seemed attainable, and I knew that I could follow them.

A few weeks later while driving, I found myself going down a street that I had never frequented before. Realizing that my daydreaming had probably led me here, I was now lost. While trying to find my way back onto the main road, I stopped the car about halfway down the street to turn around and noticed a small cottage with a "For Sale" sign beside me. Feeling as though the universe brought me here, I stopped the car and stared at this little gray cottage. From that second on, I visualized what it could look like if remodeled using my personal sense of taste. Calmly, I wrote down the name and telephone number of the Realtor. I was drawn to this little gray cottage, as it seemed to be calling out for my attention. A sense of happiness that I hadn't felt for a long time engulfed me, and I knew that this was the cottage I had dreamed about.

When I arrived home, I called the Realtor to set up an appointment to see the cottage. Although I had to cancel a few times since I didn't feel well enough to attend the showing, I was still determined to get there sooner or later.

When the time finally arrived where my strength allowed me to view the cottage, I was so excited by its charm as I stepped inside. Stepping down into one of the adorable bedrooms, I knew that this was the perfect match. When I gazed out the kitchen window, I saw two doves sitting together on an old tree stump. From that moment on, I was positive that this was going to be my cottage, especially since it was even in my price range. Decorating and gardening were my most cherished pastimes. I wondered if having a home to be devoted to would also help me regain my health.

20

A Home

A sense of pride and gratitude now filled my once empty heart as I stood outside of my adorable cottage after the move and the remodeling had begun. Traffic would often stop on the street, and people would roll down their windows to tell me that they thought the cottage was one of the cutest they had ever seen. With my energy level still too low and feeling too weak to get up to walk over to talk or personally thank them for their compliments, I could only nod my head and smile, while sitting outside on one of the Adirondack chairs purchased for the garden.

I was now seriously thinking of how wonderful it would be if I could begin a business remodeling older homes. I could only imagine the enjoyment I would have during the process of finding, purchasing, and restoring them. However, with my health still waxing and waning, this thought was only a fantasy—a mere figment of my imagination, for the energy necessary to begin such a venture required more than I could even dream of having at this point. Again, feeling that the answers for my troubled health were still an eternity away, I had to face the stifling fact that it was not possible to have a career.

After owning this property for seven months, my health began to decline rapidly. More days than not left me totally bedridden. All of my debilitating symptoms were in full-blown proportions again, raging against my fight for survival.

I now wondered what caused my health to be going downhill again as I pleaded with God to take this curse away. Why was this happening to me at this time when I felt that the purchase of a precious home would turn my life around for the better? What could I be doing differently now? What could possibly be bringing this on?

I knew that I was concerned about the remodeling contractor that I hired. I was investing more money into the house than previously estimated. As one item was being fixed, another would break. It seemed like new repairs were always needed. Interior design styles would be used that I couldn't accept. When I requested that it be changed, I was charged for the alteration again. I speculated that he might be incompetent or working only for his advantage rather than my benefit. With my brain fog preventing me from thinking clearly and too fatigued to take charge, I believed that the contractor couldn't have anything to do with my health deteriorating once again.

I can't begin to relate how confused I was because now I suffered from painful muscle spasms and pressure around my kidneys. I became so frightened.

21

Psychic or Psycho

I knew that I had hit rock bottom when I started seeing a psychic for the answers to my fruitless existence and incessantly poor health. She believed that my health problems were due to depression and fear. She also told me that I was stressed and anxious about money. My condition left me so weak and at a complete loss. I felt so pathetic as I searched for someone to trust and have faith in. Far too weak to fight, I continued on my search for the reasons of my debilitating condition.

After my first visit, I felt that the psychic was the one who was put in my path as my savior. She seemed so concerned and sympathetic to my dilemma at overcoming the chronic fatigue.

I would visit this psychic regularly, chiefly because she seemed to want to focus on a cure for me. I felt that she was truly concerned about my welfare and that she was absolutely going to try to help me.

Cunningly, she read the anxiety I felt due to my financial circumstances and knew that I was concerned about my monetary investments and the remodeling of the cottage. When someone doesn't feel well, they often doubt their own actions. She could see that I was not comfortable with the investor that I had been using to make money with the savings that I had been left with after my husband's death and the amount of money that I was using to remodel my cottage. I had cause to believe that my choices weren't proper.

When one doesn't feel well, why would they think that they could make the right decisions? If one feels poorly, one thinks the same.

I was confident that she was right about her curative abilities, and I totally trusted her. She promised she could fix all my troubles, and with my problems being cured, I would surely be well. She wanted me to do one final thing and not get stressed about it. The promise that she gave me of finding a cure was my last ray of hope and what seemed like my only chance to be well, at last.

She told me that there was one last thing that I needed to do immediately to cure myself and that she was the one who could help me with it. She told me that I should not stress about what she wanted me to do and trust her completely. Money would soon start flowing freely into my life after I began following her instructions, thus leaving me totally stress-free. Of course, desperate, fatigued, anxious, and uncertain of my actions at this point, I put my life into her hands.

The psychic told me that I should bring her two thousand dollars the following day. I wanted to know what she was going to need this money for. She told me that she was one of the few psychic healers who knew about the powers of some very rare, special crystals and also one of only a few people, who had the opportunity to buy them. Reassuring me that this price not only included the purchase price but the miscellaneous expenses, she stressed that it would take many hours, both day and night to work their therapeutic powers to heal me. I finally had found someone who cared about me. My spirits were once again lifted, just to think that an end was coming to my misery.

She also wanted to help me with my investments and told me that she understood the concern and anxiety that I had with my present investor. I was led to believe that in her line of work, she was given the opportunity to meet many people, and with her gifted psychic abilities, she instinctively knew who was helpful and who was not to be trusted. She said that she knew of one of the best investment specialists in our town and that he had helped many people reach their financial goals.

I was told that it would take about ten days for her to reach the investor. She wanted me to bring the two thousand dollars immediately, for the magical healing powers of the crystals needed at least ten days to work. I was sure to make an appointment for the following day to deliver the money to her because I felt that she was my new best friend and wanted to start working on my health right away.

When I arrived the following day, she took me into her office immediately, telling the others in the waiting room that I was in need of her immediate help. I felt so important. When I walked into the office, she told me that she was fortunate to have reached her investor yesterday and that he understood my situation and wanted to help me. He could easily triple the amount of my investment in two years and make my life so much easier. After calling him on the phone, she told me that he would arrive shortly. I was asked to sit in the waiting room until he arrived so she could meet with her other clients.

When he drove into the parking lot in a Mercedes, she called me back into her office. He appeared to be such a stunning professional gentleman, dressed in a stylish black suit by Ralph Lauren with diamond cufflinks, a finely crafted tie, and expensive black leather shoes. He had the appearance of a man who knew how to make money, and I trusted that he knew what he was talking about.

I went to his plush office overlooking the bay the following day for one more meeting. At this time, I was convinced that he would be my hero and that the psychic had put me into good hands. Not wanting to waste any time, I immediately transferred my entire savings over to him so that my investment could start earning money right away. He went out of his way to walk me out of his office to my car, stopping by the pier to show me his yacht. I was even more certain that I was finally placed in the right direction on a path to both financial security and physical healing.

Two months later, I wanted to add a built-in swimming pool to the yard of my cottage for my children to enjoy. I decided to call the investor to withdraw the money for this purpose. I was also curious as to why I had not received my monthly dividend check. I tried to call the office several times in one week to no avail. I was never able to reach the investor or even leave a message on his answering machine. I sent a friend over to his office to try to meet with him. She told me that when she entered the building and reached his office door, it was locked. No one was found at his office; even his door sign was gone.

I called my attorney immediately and sent him all my paperwork. I was told that there was not much that he could do for me because I had invested in unregistered stocks. Now I realized that I had been seriously taken advantage of by a professional crook. I blamed this painful mistake on my chronic fatigue for it had left me too powerless to be able to think clearly.

When I went to confront the psychic about this situation, she was nowhere to be found, either. It seemed that she left town just as I was discovering that the investor she wholeheartedly recommended was nothing but a fraudulent and a common crook. I realized that she never really thought about how much she could help me but rather how I could benefit her financially. I was an easy target for her. She could see right away that her scheming methods could overpower me, making her wealthier while leaving me penniless. I wasn't aware that psychic reading was just a form of manipulating a client.

Now the only income that I had was the meager amount that my son was receiving every month from his deceased father's social security benefits. Here I was, too sick to work. Not only had I lost my health, but I had also lost my entire savings, and soon I was about to lose the roof over my head because I didn't have enough of an income to pay the mortgage. At this point, I couldn't afford the necessity of having live-in help. This was nothing compared to the trauma of telling my oldest daughter that she now had to drop out of college during her first year. Fortunately, the following year she was able to get a scholarship. My disease was playing a tragic game of dominoes with my life. One tragedy followed another.

I FEARED THE TRUTH UNTIL I SAW THE UGLINESS IN LIES!
—Unknown

22

Holistic Medicine

I was becoming very ill again. Just thinking of where I was going to live was a stressful experience. The thought of winding up homeless would make even a healthy person ill. However, I was too sick to care if I had to sleep on the street. The uncertainty of whether I was going to live or die and the invariable worry about the welfare of my three children kept me stressed and extremely insecure.

The body tremors were starting up again. Unbelievable body and joint pain besieged me. All I could eat was plain boiled spaghetti and yogurt because my stomach and intestines were becoming increasingly tender and painful. I gave into the doctor and permitted him to prescribe Lortab in liquid form, a pain medicine to relieve the soreness and tenderness in my intestines and stomach, being I couldn't live with this pain any longer. While in such pain, I often caught myself gulping the bottle of medicine down like soda pop. I was also prescribed various types of antacids and medications for ulcers that caused even more pain in that area, as well as nausea. This was undeniably a vicious cycle that I had to endure.

I now heard of a Chinese doctor who had just opened a new office in a holistic treatment center in town. Everyone was talking about how well his methods worked at finding the root cause for certain ailments. I made an appointment to see him.

On my first visit, he recommended that I have a hair mineral analysis test. This was the first time that I had ever heard of this type of test. He was a quiet man and did not explain much, so I had to press him for more information about the reason for this type of testing.

The doctor could see that I was very apprehensive about this test when I asked him to please explain the validity of it. I was now so hesitant of spending any more money on any unnecessary things because I knew that my savings and finances were gone.

He told me that a small amount of hair would be taken for the analysis because I was most likely extremely toxic. The test would reveal what types of metals and other substances were in my body causing the toxicity. He convinced me that this was something that I needed. He also recommended having some blood work. I couldn't afford all of the testing required as we were now living in poverty. He could understand my reasons and went ahead with the hair analysis test only.

After the results of the test came back to the office, I was called in to discuss the results. The doctor showed me that my mercury level was dangerously high, at the top of the chart. There were also higher than normal levels of aluminum and nickel. I listened intently, but I didn't feel well enough to answer any more questions on that day. The doctor was very quiet and didn't act like this was anything to be concerned about, *mentioning that the mercury could be coming from my silver fillings.* This really left me even more befuddled because I had never really worried or given thought to the composition of my fillings or had even suspected that mercury could be found in them.

This doctor also asked me if I ate a lot of canned foods, considering that this must be the source for the aluminum. This was also nonsensical to me. I had grown up on a farm and was raised on fresh fruits, vegetables, and meats. If at all possible, I never used canned foods since I had never had the chance to become accustomed to them. Never did I want to rely on canned products for food, feeling that nutrition was of vital importance in the promotion of good health, which had eluded me for over fourteen years. After the consultation was over, and the doctor had finished reading all the results of my hair analysis, he recommended that I obtain vitamin C intravenously to help cleanse my toxic liver.

I thought about the fillings in my teeth for a while, wondering if the doctor might possibly be on the right track, for I had never suspected that they could be the cause of my critical illness. I had never thought about the phone call that I had received a while ago from my friend in California telling me about the findings and research that he had read regarding the harmful effects of silver fillings. Sick and overwhelmed, I surely had short-term memory loss, as well. Why had I forgotten about the phone call from my friend warning me about the harmful effects of silver fillings? I couldn't believe that my fillings could ever be capable of making me deathly ill. I was totally convinced that this was just another insignificant theory to take me on another wild goose hunt or lead me down the wrong track once again. Once again, I had lost my confidence and trust in doctors!

IT MAY FEEL LIKE AN ENORMOUS RISK, BUT TALKING HONESTLY
ABOUT THE SITUATION IS THE KEY TO HEALING.

—Unknown

23

The Nightmare Continues

I started getting the vitamin C intravenous solutions once a week, as that was all that I could now afford. Fortunately, the Chinese doctor charged me only half the price for them. He could see the desperation in my face. After a few weeks, I couldn't take these treatments anymore. I felt badly because I knew that this doctor wanted to help me, but the pain in my veins as he placed the needles into my arms was unbearable besides the fact that it would take an average of six times before he could inject the vein properly. I must say that the good doctor on Marco Island was the only doctor that could easily get the needle into my arms veins correctly. For the next few months, thoroughly bedridden, I wondered if I was going to die. My youngest daughter would sit by my bedside when she wasn't working or in school, holding my hand to comfort me. I could see how frightened my precious seventeen-year-old was; but little did she know that I was even more afraid for her. What would become of her or my other children if I were to die at such a crucial time in their lives?

I still kept my health problems a secret from my family because I knew that they would admit me to the nearest hospital for more testing. I had just about given up hope of a cure, and I wanted to die at home.

Now I merely existed inside of my solitary *living nightmare*. My fifteen-year-old son had to be rushed to the hospital one evening. His heart was uncontrollably racing while he suffered with high levels of anxiety. When the ambulance arrived, I was unable to go with him since I was unable to get out of bed. My condition had left me much too weak to stand up.

My daughter went to pick him up from the hospital after she arrived home from work. She was told that his problems were due to trauma caused from his mother's appalling health. This did make sense to me.

A few weeks after this incident, his basketball coach called to tell me that there was definitely a problem with my son. He had stopped performing as he used to. I tried to talk to my son, subsequently feeling guilty and blaming myself for all of his troubles. He told me that he just felt too weak to play and that his stomach was bothering him. I felt that my illness was unfairly upsetting my family.

Soon he was unable to go to school or play basketball at all. I was now sure that I was the cause of my son's tribulations. Even though the school provided him with a full-time tutor, he was unable to concentrate and had become severely depressed. He locked himself in his room, only coming out to go to the bathroom. Eventually, the fear that he might take his own life made my depression and anxiety catapult. I was at a complete loss due to my ailing condition and knew that I couldn't take charge of this situation. This went on for months when he also started to complain about body aches and pain. I was really frazzled now and continually wondered if my illness was contagious, or something in the home was the cause. My daughter called the County for an inspection to see if they would test our home for radon, mold, and lead contamination since it was nearly fifty years old. However, the results of the testing showed that our house was free of lead, radon, molds, or any other pollutants. Still in a state of uncertainty and confusion as to what was causing this miserable situation, I kept my faith that a solution would soon arrive.

Now I was no longer able to pay for the mortgage on my home. Fortunately, I was able to sell it and break even. We had to move into an apartment with my daughter's boyfriend. My daughter and her friends did all the work involved with the moving. Now my son and I had to share a room; but at this point, we were too sick to care. We could only muster up enough strength to move from the bed to the bathroom.

Since the apartment was so very small, and there was no room for any storage, I decided to have a yard sale. Of course, my daughter and her friends had to take charge of this situation as well. It was probably one of the best house sales in the area. I had to let go of my most treasured belongings, including my collection of Hummels and other antique knickknacks and furnishing, which I had managed to hold on to for years.

The only positive outcome of this painful moving sale was that I had some money to begin the intravenous treatments of vitamin C that the Chinese doctor so highly recommended. After several treatments, I was able to sit up for short periods of time and eat small portions of boiled chicken. This was a big improvement for me because this was the first time I could eat meat since I had stopped the IV treatments.

My battle continued. I was now sensitive to chemicals of any kind. I couldn't tolerate the smell of bleach, and even the aroma of hand soap made me squirm. My insides would feel like they were going to explode when I would smell certain items that I had once used daily. I now had to send my daughter to the health food store to purchase just about everything.

One morning, as I was putting my watch on, I noticed that my hand and arm were yellow, and upon further inspection I could see that my whole body had the same yellowish color. I went to the Marco Island doctor immediately. He wanted me to submit to further testing because he could tell that my liver was swollen and not functioning properly. He conjectured that I might be stricken with hepatitis or possibly had the beginning stages of sclerosis. I was also continually losing weight at this time. I had no medical insurance and certainly not nearly enough money to permit the doctor to perform these tests.

24

Natural Awakenings!

My daughter was now taking a lot of time off from school because she was too afraid to leave me alone. I also depended on her to drive me to the IV treatments for the infusion of vitamin C. At the time of life when most teenage girls are socializing, enjoying their friends, or optimistic about their future, my daughter had the responsibility of caring for an invalid mother and sick brother. She was forced to work part time to support herself and her family while most likely feeling as if her life was robbed of all her childhood dreams and comforts.

While going out of the front door of the local health food store, my daughter noticed a magazine stand with a sign that said FREE. After living with a mother who had become destitute and as poor as a church mouse, seeing anything that said FREE was like spotting a red flag. This caught her attention immediately. She grabbed two of the booklets setting on the stand and brought them home to me. She was hoping that I might find something that might be helpful to me. The magazines were called *Natural Awakenings* and *Healthy Living*. I read through the magazines several times since there wasn't much else to do while in bed all day. I found some very interesting articles like "Natural Home" and "Earth-Friendly Gardening." Not only did these commentaries catch my eye, the many advertisements detailing the numerous organic products that were for sale was also rather appealing to me. However, these articles did not reveal anything that I was unaware of or new to me.

25

All in My Head?

With not much else to do, and having read every book and magazine in my bedroom at least once, I kept on picking up the *Natural Awakenings* publication. As the week went on, I read an ad about computron testing. I thought that I had received every test ever invented, but I was not familiar with this one nor had I ever heard of it. For some reason, I was drawn to this article and decided to show it to my daughter. She insisted that I call and get more information. I felt as though I had nothing to lose, so I called the next day.

Weeks were becoming more like days, and time seemed to be slipping away from me. I often contemplated that my life was coming to an end soon. I got in touch with the office of the place that offered the computron testing and received information from a counselor over the phone. The practitioner said that the testing was done with the use of a computer that would reveal and make an assessment about the condition of my health. The computer could determine the pathology present and the functional root causes behind a disease. Individualized treatment plans could also be developed to aggressively treat the root causes. This sounded too good to be true. I was worried about spending more money on a test that could turn out to be another bogus, far-fetched scheme, predominantly because I was scraping the bottom of the peanut butter jar, so to speak. I booked an appointment anyway and asked my daughter to drive me to the office, which was a forty-five-minute ride. I had to lie down in the back seat of the car for the entire trip since I was too sick to sit up.

When I arrived at the office, the doctor asked me a few questions. He wanted to know, basically how I was feeling at this time. I couldn't even describe the pain in the pit of my stomach. It felt as though my intestines were on fire as I sat shaking in front of him.

He hooked me up to a computer. The testing was totally painless and reported the results in just a short time. Surely, I thought this was another waste of my time and money. The doctor turned from the computer and said, "Your teeth are poisoning you!" I am sure that he could see the disbelief in my face. I couldn't imagine what he meant by this. I had spent a fortune on restorative dentistry over the years.

The doctor tried to clear up my skepticism and went on to tell me that the amalgam fillings and crowns in my mouth were the cause. My fillings were composed of silver and mercury, while the crowns were only porcelain on the outside, with nickel and aluminum on the inside. He believes that these metals are highly toxic to humans and that most people are highly allergic to them.

I always believed that possibilities are infinite with an open mind. My cynicism slowly diminished as he continued to carefully explain why I was so ill. He told me that every cell in my body was inundated with toxins from the silver fillings and other metals in my mouth and that they were continually eating away at my stomach and intestinal lining. I still could not understand how my teeth could be poisoning me. How could the American Dental Association and the Federal Drug Administration allow this to happen?

The doctor informed me that silver fillings are approximately 50 percent mercury. Chewing, grinding, brushing, and the normal corrosion of metals increase the release of mercury vapors into the body. These toxic vapors consist of elemental mercury and mercury ions. While 80 percent of the vapors are absorbed through the lining of the lungs, the rest escape into the arterial and venous blood, lymphatic system, and nerve fibers. When I told him that some of my fillings were at least thirty years old, he told me that these older ones could be the most hazardous, possibly leaching the most toxins. After the doctor's explanation, I had the vision of poisons trickling out of my fillings into my mouth and then into my body since the mouth is the beginning of the digestive system.

I still doubted the doctor's explanation, thinking that he had created the worst scenario for a layman like me. I became paralyzed with fear from his chronicle about the poisonous silver fillings. I could see that he could tell that I was shaken and puzzled by his assumptions. I didn't believe that he was seriously familiar with what he was talking about and believed that he might very well be another swindler placed in my path to test my sanity. The last thing he said to me before I left his office was, "If you are unsure of what I am telling you, I highly suggests that you read *It's All in Your Head* by Dr. Hal Huggins.

I purchased the book and read it from cover to cover. Suddenly, everything that he had said made sense to me. I had never really thought about the exact materials that were used in my dental fillings or crowns. After reading the book, I realized that this was a very essential and valuable gesture! Could the use of poisonous and toxic metals in dental work be the negligence of the American Dental Association?

I also had never suspected that nickel and aluminum filled the inside of my crowns. The dentist told me that he was using porcelain crowns. Could it be that the dentist wasn't concerned about my life? Did he want me to suffer for over fourteen years with both mental and physical pain? Did the dentist really not know any better? Would somebody in the medical field take a chance of using poisonous substances that could be potentially fatal?

All these questions boggled my mind. The book revealed that any dentist, who mentions that mercury might be a hazard, is liable under the American Dental Association's commandment of ethics and could lose his license. This explains why not a single dentist had ever told me that my fillings contained the poisonous metal mercury.

26

A Cure for All Diseases!

I wanted to read more on the metals used in the practice of dentistry. My curiosity was greatly increased by the book, *It's All in Your Head*. I soon found the paperback called *The Cure for All Diseases* by Dr. Hulda Clark. I had actually purchased this book because I was attracted to the title, not realizing at the time that she had a chapter on dental metals and mercury. There was no turning back after reading this book. I now felt that these doctors were speaking the truth. UNBELIEVABLE, SHOCKING AWARENESS!

I reminisced and remembered the events and episodes of my life before I started to get sick. Of course, I had the usual childhood diseases like chicken pox. As a young girl, I was strong enough to easily get over it. My immune system was probably functioning normally during this time. I remember having energy and vitality. While growing up on a farm in upstate New York, the cold was never a problem for me, and I enjoyed playing in the snow with my friends. If confined to the house, I would always find activities to keep myself busy. I never scoffed at helping anyone or doing any chores for my family.

I had my first dental check-up when I was nine years old. During this visit, the doctor needed to do some minor work for me. I only needed a couple of silver fillings at this time. A year later when I turned ten, I developed asthma and was bothered by recurring sore throats, including repeated respiratory infections. I had never considered that the beginning of my regular dental visits was the beginning of the habitual problems with my health.

Even though I had a pleasant life as a teenager, I started getting depressed. Being the youngest of four children, my parents were very caring, sometimes doting on me. We were financially secure and never had to do without. My father was active in politics in the town, and I had the opportunity to meet many interesting people. Living on a farm was also fun, and I always had some responsibilities that I cheerfully tended to.

I was very popular in high school and can remember dating the most attractive boy in the small school. Many girls confided in me and told me that they envied me. Why was I getting depressed at this time without a reason? My gym teacher was also very confused by my behavior at this time since I was having a hard time keeping up in sports activities, which at one time had been the highlight of my day at school. He couldn't understand why I couldn't run faster. My chest would tighten up, and I would become winded so quickly.

After this time, whenever I went on bike rides or hikes with my friends, I would feel faint and could hardly breathe. The cold weather started to bother me, and I seemed to catch every cold or flu bug that came around. At the age of seventeen, I developed asthma and received regular inoculations to relieve it.

When my youngest child turned one, I had the time and money to receive extensive dental work, both corrective and cosmetic, including root canals and crowns. I also made it a practice of having regular cleanings and can remember having a deep scaling to remove tartar and plaque that had formed around the roots of my teeth. It was shortly after this time that I became very sick, and the chronic fatigue became a serious problem. After investigating the effects of the metals and other materials used in my mouth, I could appreciate the reason for my increasingly poor energy level and ill health.

When I first read the book *The Cure for All Diseases*, I surmised that my immune system had probably been suppressed since the age of nine. Forty years of having toxins poisoning the cells of my body was a long time. I never smoked, didn't care for the taste of liquor, nor tolerated alcohol. I am sure that good hygiene, including my belief in a healthy diet and proper nutrition all my life, kept me from dying.

Now I understood why the vitamin C and multivitamin IV solution was not an antidote for the toxins that had been attacking my body every minute of the day since I was first exposed to them through the mercury in my fillings. The vitamin treatments couldn't have cured me of the chronic fatigue syndrome nor have even arrested the condition because I still had the mercury-silver fillings and the metal crowns in my mouth. They could only disguise the toxicity of the metals from my body.

I could now see the connection between the sudden and complete relapse of my disease after I had the extensive cleaning of my teeth. The dentist used pumice to clean my teeth, thereby scraping the already corroding amalgams, thus increasing the release of mercury into my system. Now the mystery was solved, explaining why the mercury levels in my body were higher.

I had blindly trudged through life for so long. Caught inside what seemed like a dark and dismal maze-like tunnel, I changed direction often, taking one path after another, only to be stopped by the same impending obstacle. It seemed as if one brick wall after another stopped me along the way. I had given up hope of ever finding a way out of this disastrous tunnel. Finally, I could see the light at the end of the tunnel, and a sense of power overcame me with my sudden and shocking awareness. What had once seemed like a freight train coming head-on to put me out of my misery was now a light, my first ray of hope. After fourteen years, I realized that the mercury used in my silver fillings and the aluminum and nickel used for my crowns were the cause of my miserable disease.

Taking charge of my life, I followed the light, which led me to seek the help of a dentist. I was sure that the dentist would understand why the fillings in my mouth were making me so sick and could correct the problem. This turned out to be another barrier to my recovery. I visited three different dentists; each one insisted that the silver fillings could have no ill effect upon my health. I was getting very frustrated and perturbed by each one's reaction to my request for a consultation and a revision of the dental work in my mouth. This was another challenge for me, never expecting that a doctor would argue with my belief. My daughter would console me as I cried daily. She urged me to keep searching for a knowledgeable dentist that would be willing to be of assistance to me.

27

Taking Charge of Your Health

Coming up against opposition was nothing new for me. I knew that I was the one who had to take charge of myself and find a dentist that was familiar with the toxicity of dental metals. Finally, I remembered the book that I had read called *It's All in Your Head* by Dr. Huggins. I had the right idea when I decided to call his office in Colorado to see if they could recommend a dentist in my state. They gladly sent me a list of dentists in Florida who had been trained under Dr. Huggins's protocol.

The closest dentist was more than two hours away, but I didn't care. I knew that I needed to find the best dentist, with the most knowledge about the toxicity of amalgam fillings and other metals. I found one who was also aware of the process of dental revision, correcting the outdated dental procedures that permitted the use of potentially hazardous materials in the practice of dentistry.

Before my first visit to this dentist, I called the business, Peak Energy Performance, which Dr. Huggins highly recommended. They performed the serum compatibility test, which read the reaction level on an individual basis that a person could have to any commercial dental products, materials, or components. The assortment of substances used in the production of crowns, dentures, fillings, composites, and cements are endless.

This is a very sophisticated blood test. It delineated the reaction level into various categories, such as highly reactive, moderately reactive, and least reactive. They sent me a kit to take to a local laboratory to have my blood drawn and mailed back to them for testing. I clearly understood that this was a very important step in the process of total dental revision, since you could have an allergic reaction to any dental material, thus affecting your immune system.

Peak Energy Performance wasted no time mailing back the results of the testing. I was very impressed with the report that they mailed to me. It was over thirty pages in length, listing over one thousand dental products, including those used in fillings, bondings, veneers, crowns, bridges, root canals, impressions, and even dentures. I was in shock when I read the details of the report and realized that I was highly reactive to a very large quantity of materials used in the practice of dentistry. Although an incredible number of dentists had never heard of the serum compatibility test, I am sure that this test is of the utmost importance in the practice of dentistry.

I believe that all dentists should request this test before they begin any dental work. If this test was a mandatory course of action when I had my dental work, I could have avoided all the serious health issues in my past.

Regrettably, when I became aware of the influence of dental materials upon my health, I was not in a position to afford the cost to replace the materials in my mouth with compatible ones, and I had to make the very difficult and painful decision to have all of my teeth pulled. My health was more important than my appearance. Fortunately, the serum compatibility test permitted the dental lab to find and use denture materials that would be compatible with my immune system. If it wasn't for the testing that I had done, my new dentures could have caused a severe allergic reaction or inflicted the continued destruction of my immune system.

The total dental revision took several months, as I couldn't handle a lot of work at one time due to health and for financial reasons. As they extracted each tooth, they would give me time to heal. After each noxious tooth was removed, so were the unpleasant symptoms that plagued my health, leaving just a painful memory. After the revision was complete, my energy was restored.

I couldn't take any pain medicine because it would aggravate my digestive system and cause more problems. I decided to use acupuncture instead of drugs for the pain from the extractions. I now highly recommend acupuncture, for not only did it stop the pain but also it made my gums heal so much faster. Consequently, I could be fitted with the dentures sooner than expected.

There is a time for silence and a time to speak!
—Ecclesiastes 3:7

28

Renewed Vitality

After the dental revision was complete, my mouth had healed, and my new dentures were in place. I felt as though I had been given a second chance at life. To some it might seem like a radical method to become well, but I had tried every test, doctor, practitioner, counselor, procedure, diet, drug, and even prayer. I never gave up hope or my faith in God that a cure would be discovered.

About two months after my dentures were made and I became accustomed to wearing them, I went to look for employment. I was able to work two jobs and even seven days a week. While sick, I could never imagine having that amount of energy. My past health problems were now just a bad dream. What a change!

The only problem that continued to plague me was the intestinal pain but at a smaller degree. I went to the doctor several times. I couldn't understand why I was still having trouble in this one area. I had such positive results in the past with acupuncture for pain that I was now particularly frustrated that even this treatment didn't work. The doctor sent me for more testing, which I had to go into debt to have done, but nothing showed up. I could only eat Boar's Head low-sodium turkey and water rolls from the bakery without having intestinal and stomach pain. I still couldn't eat any fruit without intestinal pain. I tried several medications without any success, as well.

This book has been cathartic to the progress of my healing. I continued reading and researching the effects of mercury poisoning and realized that there still has to be minimal amounts of toxic metals left in my stomach and intestinal area. The doctor agreed with me.

The only method that I knew of that would remove these metals was chelation therapy, which is specifically designed to remove metals. I decided that I would need this therapy to help remove these toxins. I knew that this method would remove the poisonous metals remaining in my body. Using the internet [www.chelate.com], one can find information about this treatment.

I had seven treatments, and although they were not that pleasant for me, I was no longer awakened in the middle of the night by excruciating pains in my abdomen. After each treatment, I could introduce more foods. After the seventh treatment, I was able to eat spaghetti with red sauce.

Chelation therapy was not comfortable or enjoyable to me, but it did heal my last bothersome symptoms. During the chelation, I became troubled by blurred vision, fatigue, nausea, and depression. I was frightened; however, I was reminded that the chelation therapy was stirring up the metals and other toxins in my body as it was removing them. Since I am allergic to these metals, my body was reacting to them as they were being removed. I must remind myself that all my recurring symptoms were characteristic of mercury and metal poisoning.

I should have realized that I would be having some kind of reaction to the substance that I am allergic to as it was being agitated and pulled from my body. By the fifth treatment, my symptoms started to disappear again. I grasped the idea and became aware that it could take varying amounts of time for each person to remove the toxins from one's body.

I learned to listen to my body. I could tell when I had cleared my body of the toxic metals. I now realized that some people can be cleared of toxins after just ten therapeutic treatments, while it can take others over thirty.

I want to share with you what I now know about my journey to wellness. You can find the best doctor, holistic practitioners, treatments, books, or medicines; but if you don't discover the cause of the ailments, nothing will work permanently.

Many, who have been tormented with chronic fatigue syndrome, have thought that the causes were due to other reasons from the one that I have discovered for myself. Many believe that parasites are the major cause of this syndrome, and I did a lot of research on this subject. I can reason that the metals in your mouth can destroy the proper levels of flora and other enzymes in your digestive system. If these important natural protectors are missing, parasites and candida are free to grow and multiply, causing many upsetting ailments.

I have heard others talk about other contributing causes for chronic fatigue syndrome, including depression, bacteria, viruses, X-rays, and environmental pollutants, such as pesticides and gasoline fumes. Some believe our diet or food additives are the cause. I have even heard that chemicals and drugs from past lives can cause this harrowing syndrome. Probably the most outrageous reason was the fusion of souls, some from a past life, possibly even grotesque appearances. These can obviously lead some people to undergo outrageous treatments including exorcism. Desperate people do desperate things. I know this from my firsthand ordeal was that there are no problems, only solutions, which kept me searching and believing that I would find the answer someday.

Now it was clear to me that my son was also highly allergic to the metals used in his dentistry procedures. I decided to have my son tested because his symptoms were so similar to mine, and he tested positive for chronic fatigue syndrome. If I hadn't discovered that the mercury had caused my chronic fatigue, I would have thought that my disease was contagious and that he had contracted it from me. Now it is clear we both received the same poisonous fillings. The serum compatibility test showed that he was highly reactive to the mercury in his silver fillings. I no longer believe that there is such an illness as chronic fatigue syndrome. Rather chronic fatigue is symptoms that are caused by *mercury* and other dental *metal* poisoning.

I found a knowledgeable dentist to perform a complete dental revision of my son's previous dental work, where the metals and other materials in his mouth were strategically removed and replaced with compatible ones. Obviously, the mercury had affected his nervous system. After being a bedridden teenager for over a year, within a short time, he was able to go to work full-time. Today, he has very few symptoms left. The strange phobias and thoughts, a racing heartbeat, and constant fatigue are gone.

I now felt blessed that I had all these awful experiences so I was able to find the root cause of my son's symptoms. Who knows what would have happened to him if I didn't?

Rest assured that it wasn't easy for me to conceive that the dental materials were making my son and me deathly ill. I hope this book gains the respect that it deserves, giving those troubled by chronic fatigue the knowledge to become well. I would like to see all people get tested to find out which materials they are highly sensitive or allergic to and replace them with compatible materials so that they, too, can be on their path to a disease-free, vigorous, happy, and healthy life.

PEOPLE WHO SOAR ARE THOSE WHO REFUSE TO SIT
BACK AND WISH THINGS WOULD CHANGE.
—Charles R. Swindoll

Life is…
Life is an opportunity, benefit from it.
Life is a beauty, admire it.
Life is a dream, realize it.
Life is a challenge, meet it.
Life is a duty, complete it.
Life is a game, play it.
Life is a promise, fulfill it.
Life is sorrow, overcome it.
Life is a song, sing it.
Life is a struggle, accept it.
Life is a tragedy, confront it.
Life is an adventure, dare it.
Life is luck, make it.
Life is life, fight for it!
—Mother Theresa

29

Crown Me

Surprisingly, when I received the results of my hair mineral analysis test, I was surprised to find that I had aluminum and nickel in my body besides mercury and silver. I found out that a regular blood test will not show any traces of mercury or other metals. I also found out that the insides of a crown are lined with nickel and aluminum unsuspectingly. Do you know what your crowns are made of? Another shocking awareness! After having the serum compatibility test, I discovered that I was highly allergic to nickel and aluminum as well.

When the crowns were removed, the teeth underneath were decayed and weakened from the high number of bacteria. I had never thought about it before, but the enamel is removed from the tooth to prepare for the crown. I believe that this causes serious and permanent damage. I now disagree with the dental theory that a crown covering a tooth will protect or strengthen it.

The serum compatibility test is highly recommended, as it can provide the proper information about the materials that will be nontoxic for your crowns.

Are your *bridges*, *partials*, or *dentures* safe for your specific biochemistry? Are they *free of metals* that you are highly reactive to, as well? You must be *informed of the types of materials* that are used in the creation of bridges, crowns, and dentures. Be sure to bring the results from the serum compatibility test with you to the dentist.

These will show the dentist which materials you can and cannot use. Did you know that cadmium is commonly used in dentures to give it the pink color? This was also news to me, and I definitely didn't want cadmium in my mouth.

30

Sensational Awareness

Materials like gold, nickel, and silver amalgam conduct heat and cold faster than tooth enamel. This is the reason for the increased sensitivity to hot and cold temperatures after a new filling is placed in a tooth. In order to reduce the thermal shock from drinking coffee and eating ice cream, a dentist will frequently place a coat of insulation over the pulp chamber where the nerve lies called a base. Dr. Huggins had discovered that the typical material used as a base, called Dycal, is known to cause the same adverse reaction in people as that of mercury. I also found this enlightening because my serum compatibility test reported that I was highly reactive to Dycal. Once again, the importance of the serum compatibility test is proven.

Previously, I mentioned that I had hit rock bottom immediately after having my teeth cleaned. At that time, I didn't have a clue as to how this could be happening to me. First of all, I had no idea that my amalgam fillings were making me deathly ill. Pumice is a light, porous, glassy variety of lava used in solid form as an abrasive and in powdered form as a polish and abrasive. It is not only used in dental polish but also in jeweler's polishing supplies used for grinding and buffing the tarnish off of metals in the fabrication of jewelry. It can also be found in nail files and callous removers. Easily one can see that this is quite an abrasive material. From my experience, I would highly recommend waiting until the toxic amalgam fillings are removed before scheduling a dental cleaning.

31

Hair Ye, Hair Ye!

There are many analytical tests, but this one was the most helpful to me. The hair mineral analysis test *reports the types and levels of metals present in your body.*

The hair mineral analysis test also provides information on the minerals that are deficient in your body. Minerals are the source of all life forms called the spark plugs of life. This test was definitely a beneficial step on my road to recovery.

A separate test can also be requested for candida, which is any of the yeast-like imperfect fungi of the genus. These are normally present on the skin and in the mucous membranes of the mouth, intestinal track, and vagina. They may become pathogenic, especially albicans, the causative agent of thrush and often severe forms of diaper rash. It is a simple and painless test.

The amount of information that is revealed about your body composition is so important. Amazingly, all it requires is a small sample of hair. I found this to be one of the most useful assessments to have done, especially if you have an unexplained health problem.

You can find out more information or locations for this by contacting a holistic doctor or an advanced chiropractic center.

I never found a blood test that could show what type and number of metals I had in my body. I have been told that mercury quickly moves into the tissues.

32

The Serum Compatibility Test

This is the sophisticated blood serum test to alert both the patient and his/her doctor of the relative compatibility each dental material has with the patient's immune system. This test provides information on the patient's relative serum reactivity to all the known dental components.

Unlike tests using electrical devices, such as Dermatron, which evaluates the body's electrical data, the serum compatibility test uses the blood serum to measure the immunoglobulins and proteins, which are capable of reacting with components and corrosion products from dental materials.

It reports the degree of sensitivity of the patient. There are three levels of reaction. At the highly reactive level, the potential for damage is high, and use of these highly reactive materials is discouraged for this patient. The moderately reactive level indicates a measured reactivity, which is the less than the highly reactive. The least reactive level suggests that most people's immune systems can tolerate exposure to these materials with little or no measurable response.

This test covers all of the materials used in dentistry, such as metallic fillings, composite fillings, crowns, bridges, dentures, cements, bonding, etc. If testing for food and other environmental substances is important to control allergies and asthma, then shouldn't testing for all of the various dental materials be considered just as imperative for good health?

For a greater perspective of how this test is formulated and the span of dental products tested, I have included a sample of my test in this chapter. As you can see, the seriousness of my allergic reaction to a vast number of dental materials is quite apparent. I could now understand why my immune system was so suppressed, causing me to have all of the symptoms associated with chronic fatigue syndrome. I don't think that it is a coincidence that chronic fatigue syndrome has so many of the same symptoms distinguished in other diseases, some involving the autoimmune system. Some of the disease that seem indicative of the same conditions as chronic fatigue syndrome are multiple sclerosis, hepatitis, AIDS, lupus, Lou Gehrig's disease, fibromyalgia, and Crohn's disease.

SERUM

1. The clear yellowish fluid obtained upon separating whole blood into its solid and liquid components after it has been allowed to clot. Also called blood serum.
2. Blood serum from the tissues of immunized animals, containing antibodies and used to transfer immunity to another individual. *(American Heritage Dictionary)*

IMMUNOGLOBULINS

Any of a group of large glycoproteins that are secreted by plasma cells and that function as antibodies in the immune response by biding with specific antigens. There are five classes of immunoglobulins. *(American Heritage Dictionary)*

ANTIBODY

A Y-shaped protein on the surface of B cells that is secreted into the blood or lymph in response to an antigenic stimulus, such as a bacterium, virus, parasite, or transplanted organ, and that neutralizes the antigen by binding specifically to it; an immunoglobulin. *(American Heritage Dictionary)*

ANTIGENS

A substance that when introduced into the body, stimulates the production of an antibody. Antigens include toxins, bacterial, foreign blood cells, and the cells of transplanted organs. *(American Heritage Dictionary)*

IT MAY NOT BE THE ANSWER I WANT, BUT I HAVE TO REMEMBER THAT IT MAY BE WHAT I NEED.

—Unknown

THE SERUM COMPATIBILITY REPORT
For
Donna Haggerty
Performed by Peak Energy Performance Inc.
48680-A Edison Avenue, Colorado Springs, Colorado 80915

REPORT FINDINGS
SECTION ONE—METALLIC COMPONENTS

<u>Highly Reactive Metallic Components</u>

Aluminum	Gallium	Molybdenum
Zirconium	Bismuth	Lead
Nickel	Cadmium	Lithium
Zinc	Copper	Mercury
Zinc Acetate		

<u>Moderately Reactive Metallic Components</u>
Beryllium

<u>Least Reactive Metallic Components</u>

Antimony	Gold	Magnesium
Rhenium	Selenium	Tellurium
Titanium Oxide	Barium	Indium
Manganese	Rhodium	Silver
Thalium	Tungsten	Chromium
Iridium	Palladium	Rubidium
Tin	Vanadium	Cobalt
Iron	Platinum	Ruthenium
Strontium	Titanium	Zinc Oxide
Stannous-Fluoride	Selenium	

REPORT FINDINGS
SECTION TWO—COMPOSITES (white fillings)

<u>Highly Reactive Metallic Composites</u>

Visiomolar	Marathon	3M Filtek P60 Post
Prisma Fil	Rembrandt	Microfill Opalux
Ketafil	Revolution	Estilux Posterior
Silux Plus	Tetric	Distalite Radioluc
Z100	Bisfil P	Encore Composite
Posterior	Charisma	Distalite Radiopaq
Acclaim	Compatit R	Compo-T Self Cure
Core Paste	Bisfil 1	IPS Empress2
Bisfil P	P-50	SaturnBuildupMATRL
Infinite	Multifil VS	Herculite XRV
Lite-Fil II	Compaley	Pertac-Hybrid
Nulite	Status	Lumavis Posterior
Geristore	Visiomolar	Hybrid Renamel
P-10	Herculite	First Light
Prisma fil	Valux	Profile
Class II	Durafil VS	Compo T Light Core
Spectrabond	Bisfil 2B	Degufill H
Bisfil M	Durafil	Estilux
Fluorocore	Heliomolar	Prisma APH

Prisma TPH	Renamel	Fulfil
Adaptic Bisco	Herculit	Occlusin
Microfil	Silux	P-30
Status	Radiopaque	LC Ultra Bond
Laminate	Microfil Pontic	Bisco Blue Core
Renamel Hybrid		
Amelogen Universal		
Aelogen Microfil Estilux		

REPORT FINDINGS
SECTION TWO—COMPOSITES (white fillings)

<u>Moderately Reactive Metallic Components</u>
There are no moderately reactive products for this category.

REPORT FINDINGS
SECTION TWO—COMPOSITES (white fillings)

<u>Moderately Reactive Metallic Components</u>
There are no moderately reactive products for this category.

<u>Least Reactive Metallic Components</u>

3M-Filtek Z250 UNIV	daptic II
Clearfil AP X	Clearfil Photo Cure
Conquest DFC	Espe Compolute
Helimiomolar Radioluc	Isopost
Post Com II LC	Prodigy Paste PRDCTS
Visiofil	Acorn
Atelitefil	C R Hybrid Composite
Clearfil FII	Clearfil Photo Post
Creation I	Bisfil II
Fastset Adaptic	Helioprogress
Isosit	Lumafine
Post com II	Sculpt-IT
Wunderfil	Adaptic-Anterior

Alert   Cervident
Lumafil

Report Findings
Section Three—Bonding Agents

Products with one or more components which are:

<u>Highly Reactive Metallic Composites</u>
Gluma-3   Syntac D/E Bond   Tenure
ProBond 3   Opti Bond   Power Bond
Syntac D/E Bond
Universal-Bond 2
Universal-Bond 3

<u>Moderately Reactive Metallic Components</u>
There are no moderately reactive products for this category

<u>Least Reactive Metallic Components</u>
Acorn   Bond IT
Heliolink   Optee Dual-Cure LUT
Clearfil Liner Bond   Heliosel
Clearfil New Bond   Pentra Bond
Bisco D-E Res Bond   Scotch Bond
Universal-Adhesive   All-Bond 2
Bisco Pre-Bond Resin   Panavia
Prime & Bond   Scotchbond
Scotchbond Primer   XR Bond
Amalgambond   Bond All
Panavia 21   Scotch Bond II
Imperva Bond   Tripton
Copalite Snap Bond   Renamel Dentin Bond

The above *report findings* are just a sampling of the many materials that I was highly, moderately, and least allergic to. The findings that are on my report are too numerous to put into writing and would most likely be of no interest to the layman. The total report was approximately thirty pages long. Nevertheless, they should be of interest to a dentist who wants to safeguard his patients' health and immune system. I have listed the other categories besides the metallic components, bonding agents, and composites that I was allergic to, including my level of sensitivity in an abbreviated form so that you may get a general idea of the sensitivity that a human can have.

Out of a total of
295 dental components used for PRECIOUS CROWNS,
I was
Highly reactive to 195 of them,
Moderately reactive to none of them, and
Least reactive to 100 of them.

Out of a total of
196 dental components used for PORCELAIN AND CERAMICS,
I was
Highly reactive to 195 of them,
Moderately reactive to none of them, and
Least reactive to 1 of them.

Out of a total of
10 dental components used for PROPHY PASTES,
I was
Highly reactive to 4 of them,
Moderately reactive to none of them, and
Least reactive to 6 of them.

Out of a total of
67 dental components used for NONPRECIOUS CROWNS,
I was
Highly reactive to 57 of them,
Moderately reactive to none of them, and
Least reactive to 10 of them.

Out of a total of
45 dental components used for IMPRESSION MATERIALS,
I was
Highly reactive to 5 of them,
Moderately reactive to 1 of them, and
Least reactive to 39 of them.

Out of a total of
22 dental components used for TEMPORARY MATERIALS,
I was
Highly reactive to 10 of them,
Moderately reactive to none of them, and
Least reactive to 12 of them.

Out of a total of
88 dental components used for CEMENTS,
I was
Highly reactive to 58 of them,
Moderately reactive to 1 of them, and
Least reactive to 29 of them.

Out of a total of
26 dental components used for DENTURE MATERIALS,
I was
Highly reactive to 7 of them,
Moderately reactive to none of them, and
Least reactive to 19 of them.

Out of a total of
3 denture components used for DENTURE ADHESIVES,
I was
Highly reactive to 2 of them,
Moderately reactive to none of them, and
Least reactive to 1 of them.

Out of a total of
17 dental components used for NONPRECIOUS ORTHODONTIC MATERIALS,
I was
Highly reactive to 9 of them,
Moderately reactive to none of them, and
Least reactive to 8 of them.

Out of a total of
11 dental components used for PIT AND FISSURE SEALANTS,
I was
Highly reactive to 1 of them,
Moderately reactive to none of them, and
Least reactive to 10 of them.

Included in the report are the respective manufacturers of the dental materials, cross-referenced by a number to the specific material that they supply. A telephone number for the company that manufactures the dental material is also supplied so that one may call for an update on the ingredients used.

YOUR CHILDREN ARE NOT YOUR CHILDREN.
THEY ARE THE SONS AND DAUGHTERS OF LIFE'S LONGING FOR ITSELF. THEY COME THROUGH YOU BUT NOT FROM YOU.
AND THOUGH THEY ARE WITH YOU YET, THEY BELONG NOT TO YOU.
—Kahlil Gibran, from *The Prophet*

LIFE IS NOT A MATTER OF HAVING GOOD CARDS...
BUT OF PLAYING A POOR HAND WELL.
—Robert Louis Stevenson

33

Protecting Our Children

After reading the information on mercury and other toxic dental materials, I hope that you are willing to protect the health of your children. If you don't, who will? Wouldn't you rather use the proper fillings, possibly having to replace them every five or six years, if necessary, than cause potential danger to your child's health by poisoning them with incompatible dental materials or metals? The degree of risk varies depending on the amount of mercury, the form, how often, and the age of the exposed person. Young children are the most vulnerable to the effects of mercury poisoning.

I can picture the dentist telling you that the filling is so small that is couldn't possibly have any effect on your child's health. If you meet a dentist who isn't willing to work with you, listen to your concerns, and accept your beliefs for the welfare of your child. I recommend that you just walk away and find a new one.

I was raised at a time when there was little research about dental materials. Ignorance is not acceptable to me anymore. Every parent should be warned about the potential possibility of dental toxicity when practicing dentistry on developing young children, who are known to be so much more sensitive to poisons of any kind. I believe that "informed consent" should be a requirement in the future for all dental practitioners and the protection of all patients. Please, do not make a life-threatening mistake with your child's health.

After years of research, the dangers from using tobacco products were exposed. People now have the choice of whether they would like to continue to risk their life by using them or even being in the same room with them.

I am not asking you to stop going to the dentist or to have all of your teeth pulled. I do believe in my heart that the manner in which dental materials are used today need to be reexamined.

Testing procedures should begin before any materials are temporarily or permanently placed into anyone's body. Our children are our responsibility. Their future and their health are dependent on the actions that we take today!

34

Foods and Mercury

Fish is a highly nutritious source of protein and one of my favorite foods. Since I found out that I am highly reactive to mercury, I did more research on this matter and found out that certain types of fish have a very high level of mercury. Be careful of shark, swordfish, king mackerel, and tile fish. Tuna is probably one of the most contaminated species of fish, as it has been known to have one of the highest mercury contents, whether canned or fresh. Skinning, trimming, marinating, or cooking mercury-laden fish will not remove the mercury content.

I am sure that you understand by now the harmful effects that mercury can have on you. If you are highly allergic, any amount can be too much. Power plants and factories commit the greatest environmental contamination and pollution of mercury. Broken thermometers can also be an impending danger. Many drugstores and doctors' offices no longer carry the mercury thermometers for this reason. It is estimated that approximately two-thirds of the thirty-two thousand pharmacies in the United States have stopped carrying these thermometers, even though the United States government continues to allow the sale of them. Some people advocate abolishing the sale of mercury thermometers. They warn that one typical thermometer can greatly harm a child who inhales it after it is broken and can easily contaminate a twenty-acre lake. Even if they never break, they eventually end up in landfills and incinerators to become an even greater environmental hazard. For information on where to discard your mercury thermometer, visit the website on the internet: www.familycircle.com

35

Benefits of Juicing

Now that my body has healed from the disastrous effects of mercury poisoning, I am able to juice regularly. I highly recommend it, even before you start the healing process. If you have sores or ulcers in your digestive system, you will probably have to wait for them to diminish before you begin juicing. My ulcers diminished slowly as the metals were removed from my mouth.

It is hard for me to explain how juicing can make you feel. You will have to try it and see for yourself. It makes me feel so pure that now my body craves it every day. I am positive that juicing will be beneficial to your health because it certainly has helped me. Many health food stores sell various kinds of juicers and have several books about the subject.

The juice of fresh fruits and vegetables contain the richest source of vitamins, minerals, and enzymes necessary to nourish your body properly. Juicing is such an important step to the busy lifestyles of today. Many doctors and nutritionists believe that your diet should consist of between 50 to 75 percent of raw foods to enjoy optimal health and energy. This is very hard to accomplish for most people. That is why juicing can satisfy most people's dietary needs. The doctor from Marco Island that I faithfully visited during my journey to wellness has written a cookbook stressing the importance of fresh vegetables and fruits to avoid diseases. Processed food does not retain the important and active nutrients.

The "Juice Man" Jay Kordich is known for his statement, "All life on earth emanates from the green of the planet." Raw fruit is nature's way of giving us life. The late Dr. Bircher-Benner, who founded the famous Bircher-Benner clinic in Europe said, "Nothing more therapeutic exists on earth than green juices."

When I was young, I never thought very much about nutrition, but my mother and father gave great nutritional advice. "Eat your vegetables!" They always ate at least two fresh vegetables at every meal that they grew in our garden. Living on a working farm as a child gave us the advantage of having fresh vegetables and fruits at our beckoning at all times.

Plants derive their energy from the sun during the process called photosynthesis. "Minerals are basic constituents of the earth's crust as plants drink them up from the soil." Enzymes and vitamins are produced in plant tissues. When we consume live food, we bathe the trillions of cells in our body with theses nutrients that are derived from plants. Don't ever stop eating raw foods.

Juice is an excellent source of increasing necessary minerals and vitamins for proper nutrition. Fiber, which is necessary in the human diet, is the fundamental substance of raw fruits, vegetables, whole grains, and legumes. It is not found in animal products or fats. Fiber is made up of elongated, thick-walled cells that give support and strength to plant tissue. These cells are the coarse, indigestible plant matter that consists primarily of cellulose, which stimulates digestion. Digestion is the body's vital process, whereby your body can assimilate and absorb the necessary nutrients while helping to flush toxins from the body naturally.

I recommend discarding the seeds of apples as they contain small amounts of cyanide, which is also a poison. The skins of oranges and grapefruits and the stems of rhubarb and celery are also toxic and should be completely removed before juicing. If produce is not organically grown, it is important to peel the skin off the products before juicing. Finally, all produce, even organic, should be thoroughly washed to remove microscopic parasites, bacteria, insect larvae, fertilizers, and pesticides.

I hope that you do purchase a juicer and use it every day; if so, you will understand its benefits. I feel plants supply a miraculous abundance of energy like no other food source on this planet. I have now discovered juicing as an excellent and inexpensive source for detoxing because of its abundant supply of minerals.

BE TRUE TO YOUR TEETH OR THEY'LL BE FALSE TO YOU!

—Anonymous

36

Making the Commitment

Have you made the decision to eliminate your constricting beliefs?

I was willing to make this commitment even though it was ever so hard to believe that my mouth was threatening my life. If I hadn't had the important testing done that clearly showed the high levels of mercury and other harmful substances that I had in my body, I probably wouldn't be alive today.

Everyone should expect to be informed of the materials that are permanently, or even temporarily placed inside of our mouths. I have consulted with dentists about their understanding of the effects of dental materials to see if there has been any research by the American Dental Association since I discovered the cause of my chronic fatigue syndrome. I am still learning that there are only a handful of dental professionals who are aware. I painstakingly researched the poisonous effects that metals and other substances can have on one's health and drew my conclusions intuitively, instinctively, factually, intellectually, and emotionally. I discovered that mercury, aluminum, nickel, and other toxic materials placed in our mouths are seriously unrecognized threats, which concern public health every day.

According to a three-hundred-page report published by the United States Environmental Agency in August 1979, toxic heavy metal is the second worst environmental health problem in America. The government has the power to set standards for the use of toxic materials. If people speak out and demonstrate to our politicians that we are no longer unaware about the toxic qualities of dental metals, standards can be reevaluated and changed.

We need to realize and take the ultimate responsibility for our health. Good health is your most valuable asset and commodity. Nobody cares about your well-being or that of your loved ones like you do. It is time to speak out and make the decisions and commitments necessary to change the ignorant and constrained beliefs of our society.

The Romans wrote about the poisoning and deaths from mercury over two thousand years ago. Surprisingly, we have known about the dangers of mercury for so long and still continue to use it in our fillings today.

37

Mercury Poisoning?

General Background

Mercury has long been considered one of the most poisonous elements known to man. Despite this, the total amount of mercury in our environment has grown to the point that chronic mercury toxicity is now an endemic disease. The amount of mercury found in human bones today is 500–1,000 times greater than what is found in bones from 300 years ago. The most severe toxic effects are in the brain and nervous system.

The US Environmental Protection Agency set 0.1 mcg/kg as the maximum amount that is "safe" for daily mercury ingestion. For an average 70 kg (150 lb.) person, this would come to 7 mcg per day. In 1991, the World Health Organization released information regarding the average amount of mercury that was being absorbed daily from known sources. It is readily apparent that dental amalgams are the chief source of mercury exposure and absorption today, and on average, they exceed the "safe" limits sets by the EPA. Some is absorbed directly from the teeth into surrounding tissues where it deposits in the jawbone or enters the lymphatic system for circulation throughout the body. Mercury can also enter the nerves, directly, around the teeth and these nerves transport the mercury directly to the brain. In addition, mercury is very volatile (turns to a gas very easily), and with each chewing action, a certain amount of mercury gas is released from the fillings. It is estimated that up to 80 percent of this mercury vapor is inhaled into our lungs, and 80 percent may enter the bloodstream, being a major source of further exposure.

Mercury binds to the hemoglobin in the red blood cells and will reduce the amount of oxygen, which can be carried in the blood, which is a major cause of fatigue. Mercury at a level of 1 part per ten million will actively destroy the membrane of red blood cells.

Effects

Mercury poisoning is the ill effect on the human nervous system and other bodily systems due to the overexposure of mercury. Mercury is a neurotoxin, meaning it affects the nervous system, which causes personality changes, nervousness, trembling, and even dementia. The effects of mercury poisoning are usually classified as acute and chronic.

Acute Mercury Poisoning. Acute exposure occurs when you are exposed to a high dose of mercury over a short period of time. Adoption of safety practices in using mercury has reduced the frequency of acute exposures. However, acute exposures can occur in a variety of situations, including when children came across mercury and decide to play with it or people breathe in high levels of mercury vapor in the air. If you are affected by acute mercury poisoning, your symptoms will usually begin with a cough, chest tightness, trouble with breathing, and an upset stomach. Pneumonia can develop, which can be fatal. If you swallow inorganic mercury compounds, nausea, vomiting, diarrhea, and severe kidney damage can occur.

Chronic Mercury Poisoning. If you are exposed to any form of mercury repeatedly or for an extended period, chronic mercury poisoning can result. Mercury's health effects include nervous system problems, kidney damage, and birth defects. There are several symptoms:

1. Gingivitis—the gums become soft and spongy, the teeth get loose, sores may develop, and there may be increased salivation.

2. Mood and mental changes—people with chronic mercury poisoning often also have wide mood swings, becoming irritable, frightened, depressed, or excited very quickly for no apparent reason. Such people may become extremely upset at any criticism, lose all self-confidence, and become apathetic. Hallucinations, memory loss, and inability to concentrate can occur.

3. Nerve damage—it may start with a fine tremor (shaking) of the hand, loss of sensitivity in the hands and feet, difficulty in walking, or slurred speech. Tremors may also occur in the tongue and eyelids. Eventually this can progress to trouble balancing and walking. It has even caused paralysis and death in rare cases.

Dental Amalgam. Silver fillings are an excellent source of mercury and other toxic metals. Dental amalgam was introduced for the first time in Paris, France, in 1832. In that same year, the first case of multiple sclerosis appeared—need I say—in Paris, France. Later that same year a new variety of leukemia appeared—need I say—in Paris, France. Thus began the long sordid history of the use of mercury ("silver") fillings (i.e., amalgams) in human beings.

Dentists now place over 100 million "silver" fillings into patients' mouths each year. Each of these "silver" fillings is actually an amalgam containing 35 percent silver, 50 percent mercury, and various amounts of nickel, tin, and other metals. The average filling contains 1,000 mg of mercury. Dentists are required to keep the amalgam material in special containers, wear gloves to handle the substance, and dispose of any removed amalgams in special containers specified for hazardous waste.

Unfortunately, very few dentists wear rebreathing masks to protect themselves from the volatile mercury vapors that pour out when amalgams are drilled. It may be interesting to note that dentists today have one of the highest rates of depression and suicide of all the health care professionals. I find it totally ironic that mercury-silver fillings are considered safe and still used in the practice of dentistry today, even though some countries, states, areas, and dentists have banned the use of mercury silver.

Today, people are more aware of the dangers of mercury, and many of its uses have been discontinued. The risk of exposure due to a thermometer breaking or mercury leaking out of a thermostat or any number of mercury-containing devices is well-known today.

38

Historic Hazards

Mercury amalgams were introduced into the United States in 1833, more than 180 years ago. They were denounced at that time by large numbers of American dentists. The opposition was so strong that the American Society of Dental Surgeons, formed in 1840, requiring its members to sign pledges promising not to use amalgams. In 1848, they actually found eleven members of the society guilty of malpractice for using amalgams. All of their licenses were suspended, resulting in such an uproar that the Society had no choice but to disband in 1856.

The American Dental Association was formed and followed this group. Dental amalgams did not have a good reputation until after 1895, at which time it is believed that the ADA supported the use of mercury.

Prior to World War II, a German chemist named Dr. Alfred Stock published many articles on the dangers of mercury fillings, and many more have followed his suit, warning of the hazards of mercury. However, your dentist may attempt to refute the information available about the dangers of mercury amalgams because he/she is under pressure from the ADA to deny that mercury leaches from fillings thus contaminating the body.

Most people are unaware that the bacteria in your mouth, streptococcus mutans, can transform mercury into methyl mercury, which is one hundred times more toxic than metallic mercury. Don't listen to or believe anyone who tells you that mercury is safe.

Most dentists need to parrot back the ADA propaganda. The ADA has published and distributed guidelines for all dentists to use when answering questions regarding amalgams. Your dentist lives under the very real threat of having his license revoked for speaking negatively about amalgams.

Little has been mentioned in history books about the little blue pills taken during the Civil War. It is a well-known fact that illness and disease caused more deaths than did the battles. The soldiers died from many different causes, but it should be noted that a commonly prescribed medication to soldiers was a concoction of mercury and chalk. This medication was called Blue Mass. Supposedly good for ailments ranging from toothaches to constipation, it was a staple of all doctors' medicine chests during this time.

A Union soldier admitted to a Philadelphia hospital with the complaint of a three-month case of chronic diarrhea was treated with heavy doses of lead acetate, opium, aromatic sulfuric acid, tincture of opium, silver nitrate, belladonna, calomel, and ipecac. The soldier died after two weeks of treatment. It is no wonder that many soldiers regarded admission to a hospital as a death sentence and would endure a great deal of suffering before resorting to that alternative. Perhaps this medication was the actual cause of some of the illnesses and deaths during the Civil War.

According to a study published in the Summer 2001 issue of *Perspectives in Biology and Medicine,* President Abraham Lincoln was also taking the medication called Blue Mass. It was commonly used for depression, anxiety, and insomnia, which probably troubled him due to the responsibilities involved with being president. Other ingredients used in the Blue Mass pills were licorice root, rosewater, honey, sugar, and rose petals. A dose of these pills contained over 9,000 times the amount of mercury that is considered safe by today's standards.

Some of the symptoms, among any, of mercury poisoning are aggression and severe mood swings. Lincoln became extremely aggressive, almost to the point of becoming violent. During this time, when Lincoln stopped taking these pills, after a friend's recommendation, his aggressive behavior is said to have disappeared. Could Lincoln's erratic behavior, then, have been caused by the pills or the mercury in them?

The terms *mad hatters* and *mad as a hatter* originated during this time period when the felting industry was flourishing. The phrase *mad as a hatter* originated in the seventeenth century. Mercury was commonly used in the felting industry. In the 1860s, and for several centuries before that, hat makers were routinely exposed to mercury in their workplaces. To make felt hats, they bathed animal fur in an orange-colored solution of mercury nitrate. This process, called *carroting* after the typical color of the fur being treated, helped make the stiff hairs more pliant, thereby producing a superior felt product. The felt could then be manipulated with steam to make finished hats of any desired shape and size. Mercury was also rubbed into the brims of the hats to make them stiff.

Many felt craftsmen actually developed mental problems and became insane. Chronic exposure to mercury caused symptoms such as increased excitability, mental instability, a tendency to weep, fine tremors of the hands and feet, and personality changes, all affecting the nervous system.

Eventually the use of solutions of mercuric acid was widespread in the felt industry, and mercury poisoning became endemic.

Danbury, Connecticut, an important center of America's hat-making industry until men's hats went out of fashion in the 1960s, developed its own reputation for madness. Regionally, these employees had a commonly recognized series of ailments, characterized by tremors and stuttering. The hat makers in Danbury, Connecticut, called their disease the Danbury shakes. The mercury felting process has been discontinued.

Tragic mercury poisoning was first recognized in the early 1950s when hundreds of Japanese people and cats from the Minamata Bay area died after eating mercury-tainted fish. Others suffered uncontrollable muscle spasms, tremors, and blurred vision, giving this unknown disease the name of the "dancing cat disease." Babies of poisoned mothers were born with gnarled limbs.

The Japanese government officially recognized that the chemical maker, Chisso Corp., was not only using mercury to make plastic but also dumping the industrial waste into southern Japan's Minamata Bay. They had been pouring tons of mercury compounds since the 1930s, causing 1,435 deaths.

A total of approximately 2,265 victims were originally recognized. However, another 15,000 people have registered with the government as victims of mercury poisoning. That number could more than double because new research suggests that it can take weaker concentrations of the deadly chemical to cause brain damage and birth defects.

A professor at the Kumamoto University Medical School who spearheaded attempts to identify what concentrations posed a dangerous level to humans believed that 20,000 more people could very easily be damaged.

The government's original benchmark for contamination had required that levels of 50 parts per million needed to be detected in people's hair. But further research has indicated that levels as low as 10 parts per million can stunt the brain's cerebral cortex, the area responsible for speaking, thinking, and voluntary movement. The research piggybacks an earlier Danish study from the North Atlantic's Faroe Islands where inhabitants ingested high concentrations of mercury by eating whale meat, resulting in serious mercury poisoning.

In 1971–72, a major epidemic occurred in Iraq in which 6,530 persons were hospitalized and almost 1,000 died. In a well-intentioned humane response to famine, several nations shipped wheat grain intended for planting to Iraq. The seeds had been treated with a methyl-mercury-containing fungicide to hold down mold growth and preserve the viability of the seeds. The seeds were also dyed red to serve as a warning, and attempts were made to mark the seeds as poisonous by painting the containers with skull and crossbones. Westerners may have recognized this as meaning poison, but it meant nothing to the Iraqis. In the face of starvation many families milled the seeds directly into flour and consumed the contaminated bread. There would have been no danger in eating grain grown from the treated seeds because the subsequent crops would contain little or no methyl-mercury. However, eating the mercury-laden seeds was a death sentence.

Accidents have resulted in several cases of mercury poisoning in Michigan during the early years of the twenty-first century. Four members of a Lincoln Park family were killed after one member attempted to refine dental amalgam in his home while attempting to recover silver. High levels of mercury were found throughout the house, including wrapped food inside the freezer. The entire house had to be demolished and disposed of in a hazardous waste landfill.

A number of children have developed mercury poisoning after playing with small vials of mercury, which they found at home or school. These children were hospitalized when symptoms became so severe that they could no longer walk. One contamination incident involved closing a school for weeks and entailed environmental investigation of residences, cars, school buses, and day care centers.

In May of 2003, a British mother of three children who resides in Los Angeles, challenged the drug companies to prove her claim that a mercury-based preservative used in a children's vaccine called Thimerosal, caused autism and its devastating disabilities in two of her three children. She sees a definite link between the alarming rate at which autism has increased along with the use of vaccinations. American children are given a cocktail of twenty-four vaccines during the first two years of their life. She believes and has found evidence that mercury can cause autism in children with existing genetic weaknesses or sensitivity to mercury.

39

Other Poisonous Dental Metals

Aluminum

Aluminum, the most abundant metallic element in the earth's crust, is not a heavy metal, but a lightweight, silvery metal. Aluminum is a strongly electropositive metal and extremely reactive. In contact with air, aluminum rapidly becomes covered with a tough, transparent layer of aluminum oxide that resists further corrosive action. For this reason, materials made of aluminum do not tarnish or rust.

It can be toxic if present in excessive amounts. Even in small amounts, aluminum can be toxic if deposited into the brain. Many of the symptoms of aluminum toxicity are similar to those of Alzheimer's disease and osteoporosis.

Aluminum toxicity can lead to colic; rickets; gastrointestinal disturbances; poor calcium metabolism; extreme nervousness; anemia; headaches; decreased liver and kidney function; forgetfulness; speech disturbances; memory loss; softening of the bones; and weak, aching muscles.

Because aluminum is excreted through the kidneys, toxic amounts of aluminum may impair kidney function. The accumulation of aluminum salts in the rain has been implicated in seizures and reduced mental facilities. To reach the brain, aluminum must pass the blood-brain barrier, an elaborate structure that filters the blood before it reaches this vital organ. Elemental aluminum does not readily pass through this barrier, but certain aluminum compounds, such as aluminum fluoride, do. Many municipal water supplies are treated with both alum (aluminum sulfate) and fluoride, and these two chemicals readily combine with each other in the blood. Moreover, aluminum fluoride, once formed, is very poorly excreted in the urine.

Intestinal absorption of high levels of aluminum and silicon can result in the formation of compounds that accumulate in the cerebral cortex and prevent nerve impulses from being carried to and from the brain in the proper manner. Chronic calcium deficiency can aggravate the situation. People who have worked in aluminum smelting plants for long periods have been known to experience dizziness, impaired coordination, and a loss of balance and energy. The accumulation of aluminum in the brain has been cited as a possible cause for these symptoms. Perhaps the most alarming is that there is evidence to suggest that long-term accumulation of aluminum in the brain may contribute to the development of Alzheimer's disease.

Cadmium

Generally considered a nonessential element for organisms, cadmium occurs naturally in the earth's crust. Pure cadmium is a soft silver-white metal; however, cadmium is not usually found in the environment as a metal. It is usually found as a mineral combined with other elements such as oxygen (cadmium oxide), chlorine (cadmium chloride), or sulfur (cadmium sulfate, cadmium sulfide). These compounds are solids that may dissolve in water but do not evaporate or disappear from the environment. Besides using cadmium to color dentures, all soils and rocks, including coal and mineral fertilizers, have some cadmium in them.

Cadmium is often found as part of small particles present in the air. You cannot tell by smell or taste that cadmium is present in air or water because it does not have any definite odor or taste. Most cadmium used in this country is extracted during the production of other metals such as zinc, lead, or copper. Cadmium has many uses in industry and consumer products, mainly batteries, pigments, metal coatings, and plastics. Nevertheless, cadmium could act as a nutritional substitute for zinc in some plants in zinc-depleted environments. Organisms can tolerate low levels of cadmium in the environment. At elevated concentrations, cadmium can harm plants, animals, and humans, affecting growth, development, reproduction, and might eventually kill the organism.

Cadmium is considered a possible human carcinogen—that is, it might cause cancer. Cadmium has no known good effects on your health. Breathing air with very high levels of cadmium severely damages the lungs and can cause death. Breathing lower levels for years leads to a build-up of cadmium in the kidneys that can cause kidney disease. Other effects that may occur after breathing cadmium for a long time are lung damage and fragile bones. Workers who inhale cadmium for a long time may have increased chances of getting lung cancer. Studies show that some rats that breathe cadmium do develop lung cancer. We do not know if breathing cadmium can affect your ability to have children or can harm unborn babies.

Breathing cadmium causes liver damage and changes in the immune system in rats and mice. We do not know if breathing cadmium harms the liver, heart, nervous system, or immune system in humans.

Eating food or drinking water with very high cadmium levels severely irritates the stomach, leading to vomiting and diarrhea. The only people who have died from drinking cadmium are people who used cadmium to commit suicide.

Eating lower levels of cadmium over a long period of time leads to a build-up of cadmium in the kidneys. This cadmium build-up causes kidney damage and also causes bones to become fragile and break easily. We know that if female rats or mice eat or drink cadmium, their litters may be harmed.

We do not know if eating cadmium affects your ability to have children or harms unborn babies. Animals eating or drinking cadmium sometimes get high blood pressure, iron-poor blood, liver disease, and nerve or brain damage. We do not know if humans eating or drinking cadmium get any of these diseases. Studies of humans or animals that eat or drink cadmium have not found increases in cancer. These studies were not strong enough to show that eating or drinking cadmium definitely does not cause cancer.

The Department of Health and Human Services has determined that cadmium and cadmium compounds may reasonably be anticipated to be carcinogens. The International Agency for Research on Cancer has determined that cadmium is probably carcinogenic to humans. The EPA has determined that cadmium is a probable human carcinogen by inhalation. Skin contact with cadmium is not known to cause health effects in humans or animals.

Nickel

Although nickel is poorly absorbed from the gastrointestinal tract, dietary exposure and exposure via drinking water provide most of the intake of nickel and nickel compounds.

Nickel occurs naturally in the environment and is the twenty-fourth most abundant element in the earth's crust. Humans can speed up this release with mining, smelting and refining, manufacturing and the use of nickel-containing products.

Organisms can readily take in free nickel ions. Humans, animals, and plants can take in biologically available forms of nickel, such as free nickel ions, and accumulate them in their body tissues.

Nickel concentrations in organisms at the upper levels of a food chain, such as fish, are generally not higher than in organisms at lower levels of the food chain, such as plants. Nickel is an essential element required by living organisms for their normal growth, development, and reproduction.

Insufficient nickel concentrations in the environment can cause nickel deficiency in organisms. At elevated concentrations, nickel can poison plants, animals, and humans, affecting their growth, development, reproduction, and survival. Nickel is not considered a human carcinogen—that is, it is not likely to cause cancer. The risk of nickel poisoning is determined by its concentration and biological availability and the duration of and type of exposure such as inhalation, ingestion, and contact.

Naturally occurring throughout the environment, nickel is present in all plant, animal, and human body tissues. Its presence is beneficial for normal biological processes at some concentrations. Poisoning occurs only at high concentrations and after sufficient exposure to forms of nickel, which are biologically available to the organism.

> Everything's okay in the end,
> If it's not okay,
> It's not the end!
>
> —Unknown

40

Other Sources of Mercury

Dental revision and detoxification treatments will remove metals from your body but there are other sources for contamination and the release of toxic mercury. The following are some examples:

1. Artificial silk manufacturing
2. Bactericide production
3. Barometer production
4. Battery manufacturing
5. Bronzing
6. Dentistry
7. Disinfectant production
8. Dye manufacturing
9. Explosives production
10. Farming
11. Felt manufacturing
12. Fingerprint detecting
13. Fireworks manufacturing
14. Fur preservation
15. Ink making
16. Lamp making (fluorescent)
17. Lead-mercury soldering

18. Paint manufacturing (for natural and nontoxic paints contact:

   - American Formulary Manufacturers in San Diego at (800) 239–0321
   - Old Fashioned Milk Paint Co. in Groton, Massachusetts, at (978) 448–6336, Email: www.milk-paint.com
   - Bioshield Paints in Santa Fe (also makes stain and sealers) at (800) 621–2591

19. Printing
20. Photography
21. Taxidermy
22. Thermometer making
23. Textile printing
24. Dental technicians

A woman whom I knew developed cancer of her palate two years after having dental implants. Neither she nor her husband smoked or drank. She believes that the implants were the cause but has yet to prove this. Knowledge of materials used in your teeth can help maintain proper health.

41

Helpful Steps for Wellness

1.   HAIR MINERAL ANALYSIS TESTING

This test will give the results to show what metals are in your body and at what levels, also what important minerals your body is lacking and at what level. If requested, can also be test for candida. If your doctor doesn't offer this type of testing, call your local holistic doctor or an advanced chiropractor's office.

2.   SERUM COMPATIBILITY TESTING

This is the first test that you should receive before any dental work is started and one of the most important tests for wellness. The test selects the safest and least toxic replacement dental materials for you. This test objectively measures the degree of reactivity of one person's serum and the separate components of a commercial dental product used in the composition of fillings, crowns, bridges, cements, dentures, etc. I learned through this test how allergic I am to certain metals and other materials in dentistry. If your dentist doesn't offer this test, contact Peak Energy Performance, Inc. of Colorado Springs, Colorado, (800) 331–2303 or via the internet at www.peakenergy. com

3. FIND A DENTIST

Find a dentist who is highly trained in dental revision, the removal of mercury silver fillings, and highly aware of the toxic effects of metals and other materials on humans!

This is a topic that everyone should become familiar with. Don't be afraid to ask questions because you have a right for confirmed consent. I believe that if you have to travel to find a dentist that you are comfortable with and confident in, your health is worth it. I had to travel a great distance to find highly trained dentists in the field of dental revision who is aware of the toxicity in dental materials, and don't be surprised if you do too!

If you have the serum compatibility test by Peak Performance, Inc., if requested, they will provide a list of recommended dentists that are trained in the specialty of total dental revision in your state or area.

It is up to you to find the dental procedures that you desire. For more information on Dr. Hal Huggins Dental Treatment Center, call 866-948-4638, or visit him on the internet at www.hugnet.com. This doctor is a recognized expert in dental revision. If requested, they will mail you a copy of highly trained dentists in your area.

Contact the nonprofit group DAMS Inc. by telephone at 800-311-6265 to receive a list of qualified dentists that do dental revision.

4. BIO-NUTRITIONAL GUIDE

This test is optional. Nonetheless, it is a blood test that will give you a complete outline of your body chemistry. Before the total dental revision is performed, this is a beneficial prerequisite.

This guide puts the frosting on the cake. It provides you with a full report of over seventy pages. This will give you an important protocol to follow for the process of dental revision, dietary changes, nutritional supplements, and a program of detoxification. The hair mineral analysis is included with this test. They will also send your blood to Peak Energy Performance, Inc. for the serum compatibility test, though this test is not included in the price. I have never had the bio-nutritional guide performed as it was not available when I needed it. For more information in this test, contact 866–948–4638.

If you have any questions, please feel free to write me at:

Donna Haggerty
9 Apple Tree Lane
Naples, FL 34112

Thank you!

RESOURCES

Allergy Resources, a forty-eight-page catalog of alternative foods, books, cleaning, and baby products. (800) 873–3529.

Bronte, L., Quicksilver Associates. *The Mercury in Your Mouth: The Truth About "Silver" Dental Fillings.* Quicksilver Press, 1997.

Clark, H. R. *The Cure for All Diseases.* Pro-Motion Publishing, 1995.

Huggins, H.A. *It's All in Your Head.* Penguin Putnam, Inc., 1993.

Jerome, F. J. *Tooth Truth.* New Century Press, 2000.

Mayel, H. *Did Mercury in "Little Blue Pills" Make Abraham Lincoln Erratic?* National Geographic News, July 17, 2001.

Moore, T. J. *Prescription for Disaster: The Hidden Dangers in Your Medicine Closet.* Simon & Schuster, 1995.

Obie, W. Talk International.com, "AAA Wellness Today," 2003.

THE MEDICAL FIELD
CAN CALL IT
CHRONIC FATIGUE SYNDROME,
I CALL IT
DENTAL POISONING!

—Donna Marie Haggerty

It is inevitable that some defeat will enter even the most victorious life. The human spirit is never finished when it is defeated…it is finished when it surrenders.

—Ben Stein

www.ingramcontent.com/pod-product-compliance
Lightning Source LLC
Chambersburg PA
CBHW051105250726
48656CB00001B/477